FAMILY PRACTICE IN THE EASTERN MEDITERRANEAN REGION

IN CELEBRATION OF WORLD HEALTH DAY 2019

WONCA FAMILY MEDICINE

ABOUT THE SERIES

The WONCA Family Medicine series is a collection of books written by world-wide experts and practitioners of family medicine, in collaboration with The World Organization of Family Doctors (WONCA).

WONCA is a not-for-profit organization and was founded in 1972 by member organizations in 18 countries. It now has 118 Member Organizations in 131 countries and territories with membership of about 500,000 family doctors and more than 90 per cent of the world's population.

Primary Health Care Around the World
Recommendations for International Policy and Development
Chris van Weel, Amanda Howe

Family Practice in the Eastern Mediterranean Region
Universal Health Coverage and Quality Primary Care
Hassan Salah, Michael Kidd

Every Doctor
Healthier Doctors = Healthier Patients
Leanne Rowe, Michael Kidd

How To Do Primary Care Research
Felicity Goodyear-Smith, Bob Mash

Family Medicine
The Classic Papers
Michael Kidd, Iona Heath, Amanda Howe

International Perspectives on Primary Care Research
Felicity Goodyear-Smith, Bob Mash

The Contribution of Family Medicine to Improving Health Systems
A Guidebook from the World Organization of Family Doctors
Michael Kidd

FAMILY PRACTICE IN THE EASTERN MEDITERRANEAN REGION

PRIMARY HEALTH CARE FOR
UNIVERSAL HEALTH COVERAGE

EDITED BY

**HASSAN SALAH • MICHAEL KIDD •
AHMED MANDIL**

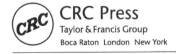

CRC Press
Taylor & Francis Group
Boca Raton London New York

CRC Press is an imprint of the
Taylor & Francis Group, an **informa** business

The authors alone are responsible for the views expressed in their contributions to this monograph and they do not necessarily represent the views, decisions or policies of the institutions with which they are affiliated, including the World Health Organisation and the World Organisation of Family Doctors (WONCA). Where authors are staff members of the World Health Organization, their contributions do not necessarily represent the decisions or policies of the World Health Organization.

CRC Press
Taylor & Francis Group
6000 Broken Sound Parkway NW, Suite 300
Boca Raton, FL 33487–2742

© 2019 by Taylor & Francis Group, LLC
CRC Press is an imprint of Taylor & Francis Group, an Informa business

No claim to original U.S. Government works

Printed on acid-free paper

International Standard Book Number-13: 978-0-367-27850-2 (Hardback)
International Standard Book Number-13: 978-0-367-27261-6 (Paperback)

Visit the Taylor & Francis Web site at
http://www.taylorandfrancis.com

and the CRC Press Web site at
http://www. crcpress.com

We dedicate this publication to the people of the Member States of the Eastern Mediterranean Region, and to the Region's health care workforce, the women and men who have committed their lives to providing high quality primary health care to the people and communities that they serve.

Family practice is the best way to provide integrated health services at the primary health care level. With an emphasis on health promotion and disease prevention, family practice helps keep people out of hospitals, where costs are higher and outcomes are often worse. Strong political commitment is essential to improve access, coverage, acceptability and quality of health services, and to ensure continuity of care.

Dr Tedros Adhanom Ghebreyesus
Director-General, World Health Organization

Contents

Foreword

Primary health care has been selected as the focus of 2019's World Health Day. The World Health Day this year falls towards the midway point between the 2018 Global Conference on Primary Health Care in Astana and the UNGA high-level meeting on UHC to be held in New York in September 2019. It offers a great opportunity for WHO to reiterate and reinforce our call for Health for all by all– with a focus on the critical role of primary health care in achieving universal health coverage. The chapters address both country-level experiences and the key dimensions which affect universal health coverage and must include – whole systems' capacity, financing models, workforce and training, and integrated needs-based care. There is emphasis on both subjective and objective domains – what patients want, how their lives and opportunities can be maximized by health interventions and accessible effective health care, and how to address population needs. There is also reflection on the modern health workforce, with appropriate use of multidisciplinary teams and modern information technologies.

The most novel thing about the monograph is its focus on family medicine and family practice – a new speciality to many, and an approach that is still being implemented in many parts of the region. Globally, the last 50 years have seen a move for all doctors to have a speciality training. For primary health care, this means training generalist physicians who can integrate diagnosis, health education, treatment, and ongoing care for patients across the life course and different health problems. The Eastern Mediterranean Region has been innovative in trying to upskill and upscale its "GP" workforce to meet the needs and opportunities of the 21st century citizen, and has taken on board the increasing evidence that family doctors with a postgraduate speciality training are highly cost-effective for any health system – because they use their skills to diagnose early, deal with multiple problems at the same time, and support both their teams and patients to work together to maximize health gains. Medical expertise is expensive, and its best use is a key aspect of affordable high-quality health coverage. For those unfamiliar with family practice, this monograph allows major insights into how countries have built this new workforce into their health systems, and how it can add value.

Of course, no one achieves anything alone. Effective universal health coverage needs appropriate financing, infrastructure, and action on the causes of ill-health as well as a strong workforce. The impact of family doctors depends on the system they work in, the conditions they work under, and the team they have around them. The World Health Organization and the World Organization of Family Doctors are delighted to see this monograph celebrate the work of so many in the Eastern Mediterranean Region, and hope that it will contribute to the future health care and wellbeing in the people of the region. Thanks to all those involved.

Dr Ahmed Al Mandhari
Regional Director
World Health Organization
Eastern Mediterranean Region

Professor Donald Li
President
World Organization of Family Doctors

Preface

We are celebrating the World Health Day "Primary Health Care for Universal Health Coverage" by the publication of this monograph for the Eastern Mediterranean Region (EMR). On 25–26 October 2018, world leaders united in Astana to renew commitment to strengthening primary health care to achieve universal health coverage and the Sustainable Development Goals. That commitment is expressed in a new Declaration which emphasizes the need to modernize primary health care and addresses current and future challenges in health systems while maintaining the core values and principles represented in the original Alma-Ata Declaration in 1978.

Universal Health Coverage (UHC) means that all people and communities can access the promotive, preventive, curative, rehabilitative, and palliative health services they need, of sufficient quality to be effective, while also ensuring that the use of these services does not expose the user to financial hardship. The journey towards UHC requires strengthening of health systems including effectively addressing social and environmental determinants of health through intersectoral action. Social health protection and equity are key considerations in UHC.

Half of the world population lacks access to essential health services, and this certainly applies to a major part of the population in the Eastern Mediterranean Region. As stated by Dr Tedros, the Director General of the World Health Organization (WHO), "implementing UHC is a political more than an economic challenge". With the 2030 Agenda for Sustainable Development, the world has signed up for UHC by 2030, meaning that a global commitment has already been made. Now is the time to transform this global commitment into national action. The World Bank estimates that 90% of all health needs can be met at the primary health care level.[1] Investing to build quality, accessible, and equitable primary health-care services is the most practical, efficient, and effective first step for countries working to deliver UHC.

In May 2016, the 69th World Health Assembly adopted a framework on strengthening integrated, people-centred health services in Resolution WHA69.24. The resolution urged Member States to implement the framework, as appropriate, and make health-care systems more responsive to people's needs. This was followed at the 63rd session of the Regional Committee for the Eastern Mediterranean in October 2016 by the adoption of Resolution EM/RC63/R.2 on scaling up family practice: progressing towards universal health coverage. In this resolution, the Regional Committee urged Member States to incorporate the family practice approach into primary health-care services as an overarching strategy to advance towards universal health coverage.

Family practice can be defined as the health-care services provided by a family physician and his/her team, characterized by comprehensive, community-oriented, continuous, coordinated,

---

[1] Doherty G and Govender R, 'The cost effectiveness of primary care services in developing countries: A review of international literature', Working Paper No. 37, Disease Control Priorities Project, World Bank, WHO and Fogarty International Centre of the U.S. National Institutes of Health, 2004, https://www.researchgate.net/publication/242783643_The_Cost-Effectiveness_of_Primary_Care_Services_in_Developing_Countries_A_Review_of_the_International_Litera ture Henceforth 'World Bank Report'.

collaborative, personal, and family services according to the needs of the individual and their family throughout the life course.

There is growing political commitment among countries of the Eastern Mediterranean Region to adopt the family practice approach to improving service provision. Despite that commitment, family practice faces major challenges in most of the Region's Member States including inadequate health facilities infrastructure, low community awareness, and insufficient technical capacity for expansion. A shortage of qualified family physicians means that 93% of health facilities are managed by physicians with no postgraduate training. The poor image of many public sector health services contributes to their underutilization. The quality and efficiency of services are further impaired by the lack of functioning referral systems and hospital networks.

There are significant challenges to ensuring effective participation and contribution of the private sector towards the achievement of public health goals. The private health sector is very active in delivering ambulatory care services in the Eastern Mediterranean Region. Up to 70% of out-patient services are provided by members of the private health sector in the Region. This needs to be taken into account in the development of strategies to strengthen primary health care and introduce family practice. The private health sector has grown with minimal policy direction and support and is rarely addressed in governments' health sector planning processes. In many countries, the private sector has emerged as a consequence of inadequate and underperforming public sector health services. Effective engagement with the private health sector for service delivery through the family practice approach is key to achieving universal health coverage.

The monograph is a collaborative effort between the World Health Organization (WHO) and the World Organization of Family Doctors (WONCA). It is the first such endeavour for the EMR. The monograph has 34 chapters, including Region-specific chapters, which highlight several EMR-relevant policy topics and how these are being addressed across the Region, and chapters outlining the current status of family practice in each of the 22 EMR countries. The authors represent a wide spectrum of global, regional, and national experts in family practice. Country-specific chapters cover primary health care and family practice development in each country with a focus on challenges, successes, and lessons learned.

This monograph is directed at policy makers, health professionals, health educators, and health students. It examines ways primary health care is being developed and improved in high-, middle-, and low-income countries, and in countries experiencing emergencies.

Hassan Salah (editor), Michael Kidd (editor), and Zafar Mirza
(Director of Health System Development, Eastern Mediterranean Regional Office
of the World Health Organization) March 2019

Acknowledgements

The idea of the book followed with this monograph was initiated in discussions between the World Health Organization (WHO) and the World Organization of Family Doctors (WONCA) during the Fourth WONCA East Mediterranean Region Family Medicine Congress held in March 2017 in Abu Dhabi in the United Arab Emirates. This is the first major collaborative effort between the two organizations in this region.

We acknowledge the outstanding and mammoth work of the 90 authors and co-authors who contributed 34 chapters to this monograph . They represent a renowned group of national, regional, and global primary health-care experts who volunteered their time and talents to this work. We enjoyed working with them and look forward to starting the next phase in developing the second edition of the monograph, due to be released in October 2020.

We thank the Health System Development Department staff of WHO EMRO who participated in reviewing the 22 country chapters, Dr Adi Al-Nuseirat, Dr Ilker Dastan, Dr Karim Ismail, Dr Mondher Letaief, Dr Arwa Oweis, Dr Hamid Ravaghi and Dr Gohar Wajid.

We thank Mr Guy Penet, and Mr Driss Aboulhoucine, the Publishing and Web Support Team of WHO EMRO, for having reviewed the Arabic and French chapters of the monograph, and our professional editors, Mrs Alice Grainger Gasser, Mrs Suzi Balaban, and Mrs Lesley Whiting.

Special thanks to Mr Hatem Adel el Khodary, Director of the Department of Administration and Finance at WHO EMRO, and to Mr Kenneth Charles Piercy of the Legal Department of WHO Headquarters, for finalizing the intricate contractual formalities between Taylor & Francis/CRC Press, the World Health Organization, and the World Organization of Family Doctors.

We thank Dr Garth Manning, WONCA Chief Executive Officer, for his continued support for this and the many other WONCA collaborations with WHO.

We thank the Japanese government for its financial support to WHO for Universal Health Coverage, and we express our deep appreciation to the EU-Luxembourg-WHO Universal Health Coverage Partnership for its generous funding to partially support this publication for the WHO Eastern Mediterranean Region Office.

Finally, we thank the team at Taylor & Francis/CRC Press for their great support throughout the preparation and publication of this monograph.

CHAPTER 1

The global movement towards integrated people-centered health services: The role of family practice

Shannon Barkley, Hernan Montenegro, Ann-Lise Guisset, Nuria Toro, Stephanie Ngo, and Ed Kelley

Despite significant advances in people's health and life expectancy in recent years, improvements have been unequal across and within the populations of countries. In addition, new health challenges are emerging related to demographic and epidemiologic shifts. The world's population is facing urbanization, migration, ageing, the global tendency towards unhealthy lifestyles, the dual disease burden of communicable and noncommunicable diseases, multimorbidities, increasing disease outbreaks, and complex emergencies, and all the while social participation and expectations are on the rise.

Having been designed to address health problems of the past, most countries' health systems are not fit-for-purpose to address the challenges of the 21st century. It is currently estimated that at least half of the world's population still lacks access to essential health services.[1] In addition to an inadequate response to financial and geographic barriers, access is further challenged in countries that continue to face problems ensuring basic inputs to the health system, including an adequate health work force and the availability of essential medicines. Even for high priority conditions, such as maternal and child health, coverage of basic services (for example, antenatal care and the presence of a skilled birth attendant at delivery) remains low in many countries.[2]

Where care is accessible, it is too often fragmented or of poor quality. Continuity of care, particularly important in the setting of chronic disease, is poor for many health conditions. Care fragmentation and disorganization, owing to weak referral systems, results in poorer outcomes and increased cost. The focus on hospital-based, disease-based and self-contained "silo" curative care models, rather than appropriately emphasizing primary health care (PHC), further undermines the ability of health systems to provide universal, equitable, high-quality and financially sustainable care. Parallel service delivery platforms, with people seeking care in both public and private sectors, can further contribute to fragmentation.

In this context, in 2015, countries adopted the Sustainable Development Goals (SDGs), including Goal 3 for health: Ensure healthy lives and promote well-being for all at all ages.[3] Target 3.8 of SDG 3 – achieving universal health coverage (UHC), including access to quality essential health-care services – is fundamental to obtaining the goal of health for all. UHC means that all individuals and communities receive the health services they need without experiencing financial hardship. For UHC services to be effective and for financing of services to be sustainable, a fundamental shift in the way services are organized and delivered is needed.

This includes reorienting health services to ensure that care is provided in the most appropriate and cost-effective setting, with the right balance between out- and in-patient care while strengthening the coordination of care across settings. Health services should be organized around the comprehensive needs and expectations of people and communities, empowering them to take a more active role in their health and health system.

PHC-orientation within health systems is associated with better outcomes that are accessible, equitable, effective, safe, people-centred care – and is therefore essential to achieving the goals for effective coverage. PHC-orientation is also cost-effective, promoting sustainability of health system financing and enabling progressive realization of UHC. PHC, with its emphasis on whole-person care, coordination and continuity is also associated with higher levels of responsiveness.[4]

Research over the past decades has identified the characteristics that are shared by high-performing primary care systems, those qualities that most ensure primary care serves its crucial function. These characteristics influence access, equity, cost-effectiveness, safety, and effectiveness of primary care: first-contact, person-centred, continuous, comprehensive, coordinated, family and community oriented, and are central to a family practice approach.[5]

Given its foundational importance to health systems, primary care has never left the policy agenda; however, in many countries, primary care still does not receive the attention, resources or support necessary to fulfil its fundamental role. As a result, too often primary care falls short of its potential. For primary care to fulfil its critical role for future health needs, reforms must address structural and financial support as well as reorient the models of health care to meet today's health demands.

Family practice enables high-performing PHC. Transforming health systems to be more integrated and people-centred, including a renewed emphasis on primary health care, can address current demographic, epidemiologic and health system challenges.

REFERENCES

1. World Health Organization and the International Bank for Reconstruction and Development/The World Bank. *Tracking Universal Health Coverage: 2017 Global Monitoring Report*. Geneva : World Health Organization, 2017.
2. Countdown to 2015: maternal, newborn and child survival. *Country Profiles*. [Online] [Accessed: January 22, 2018.]
3. United Nations. Sustainable Development Goals: 17 Goals to Transform our World. [Online] [Accessed: January 22, 2018.] http://www.un.org/sustainabledevelopment/health/.
4. World Health Organization. *People-centred and integrated health services: a review of the evidence*. Geneva : WHO Press, 2015. WHO/HIS/SDS/2015.7.
5. Starfield B, Shi L, Macinko J. *Contribution of primary care to health systems and health*. Millbank Quarterly, 2005; 83: 457–502.

CHAPTER 2

Scaling up family practice: Progressing towards universal health coverage in the Eastern Mediterranean Region

Zafar Mirza, Mohammad Assai Ardakani, and Hassan Salah

The World Health Assembly (WHA) Resolution 69.24 on "Strengthening Integrated, People-Centred Health Services [IPCHS]" was endorsed by the 69th session of the World Health Assembly, held in May 2016. The IPCHS resolution urged Member States to implement, as appropriate, the framework of action and make health-care systems more responsive to people's needs. In the Eastern Mediterranean Region Office of the World Health Organization (WHO), this strategy is operationalized on the level of primary care service through the Family Practice (FP) programme. The Eastern Mediterranean Regional Committee, at its 63rd session in October 2016, adopted the Resolution for Agenda item 4(a) "Scaling up family practice: progressing towards universal health coverage". The resolution urged Member States to incorporate the FP approach into primary health-care services as an overarching strategy to advance towards universal health coverage.

Family practice can be defined as the health-care services provided by a family physician and the members of his/her team, characterized by comprehensive, community-oriented, continuous, coordinated, collaborative, personal, and family services according to the needs of the individual and their family throughout the life course. Family practice, as a first point of contact with the health service, is key to delivering effective health services and improving health through holistic approaches that ensure continuity of care. Family practice can deal with the majority of the health and health-care needs of individuals, their families, and their communities.[1]

The terms "family practice" and "family medicine" are often used interchangeably in the literature. The latter is defined as the specialty of medicine concerned with providing comprehensive care to individuals and families, and integrating biomedical, behavioural, and social sciences. As an academic medical discipline, it includes comprehensive health-care services, education, and research.[2]

The scope of services delivered by family practice requires a multidisciplinary team and the spirit of family practice emphasizes a team approach to service delivery. The composition of the team may vary among countries depending on the service package, structures, resources, and availability of human resources, but should include at least a family physician and a nurse.

The evidence supports the contribution of a well-trained family practice team to improving access to quality care[3]. The family physician and nurse are the backbone of family practice. However, there is a worldwide shortage of family physicians, with an acute situation in the Eastern Mediterranean Region.

As well as improving training capacities, labour market dynamics should be considered in attracting and retaining health workers to work in family practice settings. Most countries in the Eastern Mediterranean Region face workforce challenges in primary care settings, especially in rural and remote areas. Thus, adequate incentives should be introduced to attract physicians to specialization in family medicine, as well as for the other professionals that are included in the family practice team. These incentives, which may be both financial and non-financial, as well as professional and personal, need to be designed to meet both the needs of communities and the preferences of health professionals.

Almost half the countries in the Eastern Mediterranean Region have already adopted models of family practice and are at different stages of implementation. Several countries have yet to evolve workable family practice models due to challenges such as a lack of trained family physicians, lack of integration of prevention and care of non-communicable diseases and mental health, and weak information and surveillance systems.

The recommended framework for action on advancing family practice towards universal health coverage consists of five major areas with actions outlined for countries and the WHO.

1. *Governance:* Health systems need to be reoriented and their capacity needs to be developed to support family practice. Governments need to ensure political commitment and develop appropriate polices, regulations, and prepayment schemes for the provision of an essential health services package through the family practice approach.
2. *Scaling up of family medicine training programmes:* To increase the number of licensed family physicians, the discipline of family medicine needs to be established and strengthened. As a transitional arrangement, suitable bridging programmes are needed to upgrade general practitioners to family physicians.
3. *Financing:* Countries need to enhance financing, undertake costing of essential health service packages, and practice strategic purchasing.
4. *Integration and quality assurance of services:* A range of well-selected, quality assured health services should be provided in an integrated manner through family practice, backed up by a robust referral system. Health facilities must be accredited.
5. *Community empowerment:* Community leaders and volunteers can bridge households to health-care facilities. Community participation in health care needs to be strengthened by building on local systems of engagement and by respecting local cultures and belief systems.

REFERENCES

1. Boelen C. In: *Improving Health Systems: the Contribution of Family Medicine: A Guidebook.* Singapore: World Organization of Family Doctors, 2002.
2. Kidd M (ed). *The Contribution of Family Medicine to Improving Health Systems: A Guidebook from the World Organization of Family Doctors,* 2nd edition. London: Radcliffe Health, 2013.
3. World Health Organization. *Quality assessment of service provision at primary health care level.* World Health Organization, 2014 (unpublished).

CHAPTER 3

Universal health coverage: Challenges and opportunities for the education of the health workforce

Amanda Howe

For universal health coverage (UHC) to have a meaningful future there must be a health workforce that is trained to work across different needs at the first point of care, with health professionals who are committed to working in primary care settings, and to meeting the needs of all people.

Whether training doctors, nurses, or other health workers, there are some core professional principles which underpin UHC – the first is the principle of *equity*, defined as *"the principle and practice of ensuring the fair and just allocation of resources, programmes, opportunities and decision-making to all groups, while reflecting different needs and requirements"*. Learning to put the needs of others above one's own, and to treat people who are very different from oneself with respect and compassion, requires very different educational approaches from the learning of technical skills or bioscientific facts.

Another is the principle of *generalism*[1] – if health workers are to address promotive, preventive, curative, rehabilitative and palliative aspects of care, they will need to gain and be willing to utilise a broad range of knowledge, even within their own subject or scope of practice.

A third principle is '*integration*' – the World Health Organization (WHO) recommends care which is integrated and person-centred[2] by which is meant a genuine intention and ability to engage with people and communities in their many unique and diverse aspects, and to work with as many different aspects of care at the same time as is feasible and effective. Learning to be person-centred rather than disease-centred is a key aspect of a modern curriculum, and again may need both different methods of learning and assessment to become embedded in the professional's practice.

And finally, the principle of '*academic analysis*', whereby the health worker routinely asks themselves why something is occurring, considers the evidence base that can be applied to the problem, and looks for ways to improve and learn from each problem in practice[3].

Working with these four principles of equity, generalism, integration and academic analysis, we can begin to see why modern health professional training needs to be different to deliver UHC.

Professional leaders and educators, with national and institutional support, have a crucial role in shifting the balance of the learning environment, to emphasise the broader context of common problems played out in all parts of society, and equipping the future workforce to be competent and motivated to address the personal and population needs of the communities they will serve. This needs a change in curriculum, educational methods, and training culture – as well as change elsewhere in the system. The Eastern Mediterranean Region has many experienced clinicians and educators, with some mature examples of universal health coverage.

Core principles behind reforms include equity; prioritising generalist practice; developing person centredness with integration of care around the individual and their needs; exposing learners at all levels to learning from real people and communities; and ensuring they understand how health systems achieve universal health coverage.

Targets may need to be set and held accountable for numbers needed entering medicine and nursing, especially for staff working in primary care and frontline ambulatory settings, so that each health system achieves the right workforce in the right place with the right skills and attitudes. It is important to consider selection criteria and the expectations of those entering the health workforce.

Also important is the need for curricula to build professional and communication skills as well as bioscientific and disease specific learning. Increased use needs to be made of direct patient contact, and of learning settings outside major hospitals.

Actions are needed at multiple levels, and momentum needs to be built, even where capacity is initially limited. Actions include advocacy, increasing the skills of existing workforce, incentivizing and rewarding innovation, and working with students, faculty, health professionals and patients to achieve the changes needed.

Risks, such as brain drain of trained health professionals from low- and middle-income countries to high-income countries, need to be tackled at the same time, and all medical specialities need to respect and support each other across both primary and secondary care.

There needs to be encouragement of those responsible (usually universities, Ministries of Health and/or Education, professional societies, and accreditation bodies) to align their programmes to the overall strategic goal of achieving universal health coverage.

REFERENCES

1. Howe A, for the Royal College of General Practitioners. *Why expertise in whole person medicine matters.* London; RCGP: 2012. http://www.rcgp.org.uk/policy/rcgp-policy-areas/~/media/Files/Policy/A-Z-policy/Medical-Generalism-Why_expertise_in_whole_person_medicine_matters.ashx (accessed 3/1/18).
2. *Framework on integrated person-centred health services.* World Health Organization, 2016. http://apps.who.int/gb/ebwha/pdf_files/WHA69/A69_39.pdf?ua=1 (accessed 14/1/18).
3. Greenhalgh T, Douglas HR. *Experiences of general practitioners and practice nurses of training courses in evidence-based health care: a qualitative study.* British Journal of General Practice, 1999; 49: 536–540.

CHAPTER 4

Proactive Primary Care: Integrating public health and primary care

Salman Rawaf, Elizabeth Dubois, Mays Rahem, and David Rawaf

The 2018 Declaration of Astana re-focused on what was declared at Alma-Ata 40 years earlier: the crucial role of primary care in attaining the World Health Organization's goal of health for all, addressing inequalities and achieving universal health coverage.[1,2]

While primary care has been associated with enhanced access to health services, better health outcomes, and a decrease in hospitalization and emergency department visits, it can also help counteract the negative effect poor economic conditions can have on health.[3,4] However, traditional primary care, as we know it, focuses on personal health care services and continuity of care. The curative "disease model" of the 1970s, still practiced in many countries, is changing rapidly. Demographic and epidemiological changes like ageing, population growth, the growing burden of chronic, noncommunicable disease and multimorbidity, along with technological advances, are driving the transformation of primary care away from the dated medical model. This paradigm shift require primary care to focus on prevention and quality of life, and encourage a proactive population management approach that targets individuals and groups that are most affected by the structural determinants of health. To be effective requires strong links between public health and primary care.

There is no perfect health system; each model has its strengths and weaknesses. But we also know that those most effective systems are those able to secure the health of the population as a whole.[5] This is impossible without universal health coverage achieved through effective comprehensive primary care focused not only on disease but also on health and how to improve it. Therefore, a strong, proactive public health function is required within primary care to protect the health of the population and that of the individual, promote health, and prevent disease.[6]

The integration of public health into primary care could be achieved through various means: relocating public health professionals into primary care settings; creating comprehensive and proactive package that include a wide range of public health interventions at both population and individual levels; primary care provided within public health settings; building public health incentives into primary care; and initiating public health training for primary care staff, doctors and nurse.[7]

Public health and primary care are natural allies and their integration should be achieved both at academic and service delivery levels. Proactive, comprehensive and integrated primary care saves lives, reduces the burden of disease and improves the quality of life. It is also an important means to improve productivity, enhance service quality, provide a seamless service and achieve universal health coverage.[8] With such strong evidence, policy change and implementation should be swift.

REFERENCES

1. World Health Organization and United Children's Fund. Declaration of Astana. Geneva: WHO, 2018. https://www.who.int/docs/default-source/primary-health/declaration/gcphc-declaration.pdf (accessed 20 December 2019)

2. Primary care: Now more than ever. World Health Report 2008. Geneva: World Health Organization; 2008 https://www.who.int/whr/2008/en/, accessed 10 October 2018).

3. Kane RL, Keckhafer G, Flood S, Bershadsky B, Siadaty MS. The effect of Evercare on hospital use. J Am Geriatr. 2003;51:1427–34. doi: 10.1046/j.1532–5415.2003.51461

4. Shi L. The impact of primary care: a focused review. Scientifica (Cairo). 2012;2012:43289. doi: 10.6064/2012/432892

5. Wanless D. Securing good health for the whole population. Final report. London: HMSO; 2004 https://www.southampton.gov.uk/moderngov/documents/s19272/prevention-appx%201%20wanless%20summary.pdf (accessed 20 January 2019)

6. Rawaf S. A proactive general practice: integrating public health into primary care. London J Prim Care (Abingdon). 2018;10:17–8. doi: 10.1080/17571472.2018.1445946

7. Rawaf S. Medico de familia na saude publica (Family physicians and public health). In: Gusso G, Lopes JMC, editors. Tratado de medicina de familia e communidade: principios, formaco et practica (Treatise on family and community medicine: principles, training and practice). Porto Alegre: Artmed Editora Ltda; 2012. Volume 1:19–27.

8. Baker R, Honeyford K, Levene LS, Mainous AG, Jones DR, Bankart MJ, et al. Population characteristics, mechanisms of primary care and premature mortality in England: a cross-sectional study. BMJ Open. 2016;6:e009981. doi:10.1136/ bmjopen-2015–009981

Health information in primary care and family practice: Concept, status, and a vision for the Eastern Mediterranean Region (EMR)

Arash Rashidian, Henry Victor Doctor,
Eman Abdelkreem Hassan Aly,
and Azza Mohamed Badr

A health information system (HIS) is an "integrated effort to collect, process, report and use health information and knowledge to influence policy-making, programme action and research".[1] HIS is one of the essential building blocks of a health system, enabling decision-makers at all levels of the health system to identify health challenges and make optimal allocation of scarce resources to achieve health improvements. A robust HIS that generates reliable, timely, and high-quality data is among several factors that enable policy makers to make evidence-based decisions.

Health data and information come from two main categories: population-based data sources (censuses, vital registration, and household surveys) and institution-based data sources (facility surveys, facility records, individual records).[2] Routine health information systems (RHIS) data, also called health facility and community information systems, are recognized as the backbone of facility-level, micro-planning, and higher-level (e.g. district, regional, national) decision making, resource allocation, and health strategy development.[3] Routine HIS consists of data collected at regular intervals in public, private, and community-level health facilities and institutions. The data provides an opportunity to study dynamics in health status, health services, and health resources.

Despite the renewed interest and significant investments in RHIS data for country-led programmes and policy making, there are major obstacles that impede the quality and effective use of RHIS data. A common concern in many settings relates to delayed submission of reports including incomplete and inaccurate data from health facilities and districts. Such data quality issues undermine credibility and compromise use of RHIS-based indicators. However, there are effective, novel, and innovative approaches, often using information technology for improving routine HIS data particularly in low- and middle-income countries. These methods have led to significant improvements in data quality by taking advantage of the available electronic data systems to enhance data collection, processing, analysis, and use of information.[4] Data quality assessments and ensuing improvement plans have also led to widespread use of routine HIS data for decision making.

Implementation of facility-based information systems has created opportunities for collection of information related to the efficacy of interventions, treatment administration, and related outcomes. When such data are collected, they can be used for a wide range of purposes, including managing patient care, epidemiological surveillance, monitoring of intervention-specific programmes, and quality assessments. Further, these data can be useful in complementing other sources of data to detect and report epidemic outbreaks.

While HISs are essential for the effective conduct of primary care and family practice approaches, countries in the Eastern Mediterranean Region (EMR) vary substantially in their methods of collection, use, and oversight of HISs. Even in countries with similar PHC prototypes, based on WHO recommendations, the HISs vary to a large extent. This may be partly because, from the start, a systemic approach was not offered for HIS implementation alongside primary care; and the minimum characteristics of an effective HIS were not defined in detail.

Despite these variations, HISs in different countries' primary care systems provide enough insight for action and some opportunities for learning. The World Health Organization in the EMR has a plan of action to improve HISs. This plan of action includes a regional framework for the collection and reporting of core indicators, a plan for improving national civil registration and vital statistics (CRVS) systems, with a focus on mortality registration and accurate certification of causes of death, and a model for the conduct of comprehensive HIS assessments.[5-6] The latter provides ample attention to the organization of national HISs, including in primary care, and it is hoped it will help the consolidation of actions to support continuous improvement of primary care systems.

REFERENCES

1. Lippeveld T. Routine health information systems: The glue of a unified health system. [Keynote address] Workshop on Issues and Innovation in Routine Health Information in Developing Countries. Potomac, Washington, DC, 14–16 March 2001.
2. Health Metrics Network. Assessing the National Health Information System: An Assessment Tool Version 4.00. Geneva: World Health Organization, 2008.
3. Mutale W, Chintu N, Amoroso C, Awoonor-Williams K, Phillips J, Baynes C, et al. Improving health information systems for decision making across five sub-Saharan African countries: Implementation strategies from the African Health Initiative. *BMC Health Services Research,* 2013; 13(Suppl 2): S9. Available from: http://www.biomedcentral.com/1472–6963/13/S2/S9 [Accessed 17 February 2018].
4. Wagenaar BH, Sherr K, Fernandes Q, Wagenaar AC. Using routine health information systems for well-designed health evaluations in low-and middle-income countries. *Health Policy and Planning,* 2016; 31(1): 129–135.
5. Alwan A, Ali M, Aly E, Badr A, Doctor H, Mandil A, Rashidian A, Shideed O. Strengthening national health information systems: Challenges and response. *Eastern Mediterranean Health Journal,* 2016; 22(11): 840–850.
6. World Health Organization. Regional Strategy for the Improvement of Civil Registration and Vital Statistics System 2014–2019. Cairo: WHO Regional Office for the Eastern Mediterranean, 2014.

CHAPTER 6

Integration of non-communicable diseases in primary health care in the WHO Eastern Mediterranean Region

Slim Slama, Gemma Lyons, Heba Fouad, Shannon Barkley, and Asmus Hammerich

Non-communicable diseases (NCDs) are a great burden in the Eastern Mediterranean Region (EMR) representing 63% of all registered deaths. This proportion is projected to increase to nearly 70% by 2030. Addressing the social and economic burden posed by these conditions requires a whole-of-a-government and a-whole-of-a-society approach in order to develop national country responses that integrate population-wide preventative measures, combined with health services able to detect early and manage NCDs and their related risk factors, by prioritizing and integrating the most cost-effective interventions, known as the World Health Organization (WHO) recommended 'best buys'.

WHO's 2016 'Framework on integrated, people-centered health services' emphasizes the importance of organizing primary health care (PHC) around the comprehensive needs of people, rather than around a singular focus of specific diseases. Furthermore, the momentum created by the Sustainable Development Goals, and the efforts being made to expand universal health coverage (UHC), are bringing a renewed focus on key essential NCD interventions to be integrated as part of a given country service delivery packages, the levels where those interventions are expected to be delivered, the health systems requirements needed to deliver them, as well as the healthcare financing mechanisms needed to guarantee financial protection and reduction of out-of-pocket spending.

A standard definition for NCD integration within PHC does not yet exist. However, it can be described as the process of embedding NCDs into PHC across all health system domains. WHO has defined the health system building blocks as:[1] leadership and governance, health financing, health workforce, medical products, vaccines and technologies, health information, and health service delivery.

For example, integration at the governance level would include strategies such as a financed and operational national NCD plan that includes a monitoring and evaluation framework. At the human resources level, integration requires strategies such as inclusion of NCD knowledge and competencies in the training, recruitment and retention of the PHC workforce, an emphasis on interdisciplinary teamwork and role allocation to ensure appropriate use of available resources based on population health needs. Importantly, some competencies and approaches might be shared across all four of the major NCDs, such as targeting their shared risk factors.

While challenges differ according to the level of resources and health systems development, a number of common challenges have been identified to NCD integration, including: lack of funding; lack of standards/guidelines/protocols; insufficient number of staff and inadequate training; lack of public awareness; insufficient availability of essential NCD medicines and technologies; a tendency to focus on curative care; and less experience in integrating early detection interventions. as well as deficient information systems to provide information on quality of care and programme performance.

The World Health Organization (WHO) periodically monitors the capacity of Member States to respond to the NCD epidemic, through a global survey, known as the NCD Country Capacity Survey (NCD CCS).[2] The global survey, undertaken since 2000, covers: health system infrastructure; funding; policies, plans and strategies; surveillance; and partnerships and multilateral collaboration. A specific set of questions assess national capacity for NCD management at the primary health care level. This provides a useful course of information to compare between the WHO regions on the integration of NCDs within PHC.

Despite the differences in health system performance and level of health expenditure, the service delivery of NCD-orientated PHC is a constraint common to each of the Member States of the EMR. The Region's PHC systems have traditionally focused on communicable diseases, other acute conditions, and maternal and child health. Primary health care was consequently arranged vertically and organized according to specific services. This structure was incompatible with the need to develop a holistic appreciation of the PHC visitor, and his or her health conditions and lifestyle throughout the life course. Therefore, a transition has begun, allowing primary health care to move away from the vertical, disease-specific approaches of the past and towards a broader people-centered care.

Integration approaches will need to be scaled up across the region for the countries to achieve the United Nation targets on NCDs by 2025. The health system approach outlined offers a systematic way to identify and progressively address the health system bottlenecks that hinder effective integration.

REFERENCES

1. WHO Western Pacific Region. Health Services Development. The WHO Health Systems Framework. http://www.wpro.who.int/health_services/health_systems_framework/en/ [Accessed 7th December 2017].
2. WHO. Noncommunicable disease and their risk factors: Assessing national capacity for the prevention and control of NCDs. http://www.who.int/ncds/surveillance/ncd-capacity/en/ [Accessed 15th December 2017].

CHAPTER 7

Family practice workforce: multidisciplinary teams

Fethiye Gülin Gedik, Arwa Oweis, and Merette Khalil

In efforts to advance towards universal health coverage (UHC), there is a global and regional trend towards implementing family practice-based primary care. However, many countries in the Eastern Mediterranean Region (EMR) not only face an overall shortage of health workers, but also face challenges in attracting, recruiting, and retaining health professionals to work in primary care settings. This has a significant impact on the availability, accessibility, and quality of services provided in primary care settings, especially in rural and remote areas.

Family practice (FP) models emphasize the importance of the multidisciplinary team as a way to deliver high-quality primary care.[1,2] The composition of the team may vary among countries depending on the essential service package, structures, resources, and availability of human resources.

Health professional education should include adequate exposure to primary care facilities and community-based training, while also strengthening skills in communication, assertiveness, critical thinking, and decision-making to meet the needs of their communities in providing patient-centered care and demonstrating inter-professional and practice management skills.[3]

Many countries in the EMR suffer from shortages, suboptimal production, imbalanced geographic, gender and skill-mix distributions and concerns related to quality, relevance and performance. Shortages are most critical at the primary care level. Countries with critical shortages of health workers may have difficulty in deploying adequate numbers of physicians and nurses to primary care facilities, especially in rural areas. In some cases, the primary care facilities will not be staffed with physicians at all. For example, in Iraq, 40% of primary health-care centres lack physicians, 84% of doctors are based in urban areas, 74% work in hospitals, and only 23% work in PHC centres.[4,5] In Somalia, only 9% of physicians are employed in rural settings.[6]

While urbanization continues to increase globally and in the EMR, 60% or above of the populations of low-income and low-to-middle-income countries in the EMR live in rural areas. Ensuring adequate family practice-based primary care will require the introduction of necessary interventions and incentives to attract health professionals to work at the primary care level. It is well known that a combination of educational and regulatory interventions, financial incentives, as well as professional and personal support may help to improve deployment and retention in primary care as well as in rural and remote areas, leading to improved distribution of health workers.[7]

These trends indicate that shortages will continue and health professionals' preferences towards specialization and working in hospital settings may be obstacles to strengthening primary care, moving towards FP models, and achieving UHC. Interventions are urgently needed to achieve specialization of doctors as family physicians and to encourage work at the primary care level.

Family practice-based primary care goes beyond training and introducing family physicians into the system. Significant attention and effort is often diverted to training and scaling up of family physicians, without enough attention paid to training the other members of the team, particularly the nursing and midwifery workforce.

Financial incentives, payment mechanisms to improve performance, better working environment, and access to adequate medicines and supplies are some important examples of system-related changes needed to ensure that the trained primary care health workforce does not leave the country or move to the private sector. System changes should influence both provider and user behavior while improving quality of services.

The family practice-based primary care model in the EMR is still fragmented, poorly staffed, and underutilized. Serious political efforts, financial investments and improving health professional education are needed to strengthen family practice-based primary care towards building a sustainable interdisciplinary team able to respond to the needs of the population.

REFERENCES

1. Rodriguez HP, Rogers WH, Marshall RE, Safran DG. Multidisciplinary primary care teams: Effects on the quality of the clinician-patient interactions and organizational features of care. *Med Care,* 2007; 45(1): 19–27.
2. Schuetz B, Mann E, Everett W. Educating health professionals collaboratively for team-based primary care. *Health Aff (Millwood),* 2010; 29(8): 1476–80.
3. Babiker A, El Husseini M, Al Nemri A, Al Frayh A, Al Juryyan N, Faki M, et al. Health care professional development: Working as a team to improve patient care. *Sudanese J Paediatrics.* 2014; 14(2): 9–16.
4. Al Hilfi TK, Lafta R, Burnham G. Health services in Iraq. *Lancet,* 2013; 381(9870): 939–48.
5. Shukor AR, Klazinga NS, Kringos DS. Primary care in an unstable security, humanitarian, economic and political context: The Kurdistan Region of Iraq. *BMC Health Serv Res,* 2017; 17(1): 592.
6. WHO. Strategic review of the Somali health sector: Challenges and prioritized actions. Available from: http://moh.gov.so/en/images/publication/review_somali_Health_sector.pdf [Accessed 26 December 2017].
7. WHO. Increasing access to health workers in remote and rural areas through improved retention. Available from: http://www.who.int/hrh/retention/guidelines/en/ [Accessed 18 January 2018].

CHAPTER 8

Current status of family medicine education and training in the Eastern Mediterranean Region

Waris Qidwai and Gohar Wajid

Family Medicine (FM) is witnessing expansion in the Eastern Mediterranean Region (EMR) at a variable pace. Progress is hindered by lack of availability of trained human resources, mainly due to a shortage of training programs and lack of support from some policy makers for the specialty.[1] There are many examples of countries that have benefited from the Family Practice (FP) model.[2] It has been recommended that 20% of all doctors in the six Member States of the Gulf Cooperation Council (GCC) should be trained as specialists in family medicine over the next 10 years, but, taking Bahrain as an example, it will require more than 20 years to achieve the target.[3]

Family medicine education and training needs to be addressed at the level of undergraduate medical education, postgraduate training, and training to build the capacity of the existing medical workforce.

FAMILY MEDICINE DEPARTMENTS AND UNDERGRADUATE MEDICAL EDUCATION

Undergraduate programs in FM are essential to serve as the foundation for the specialty. Medical students need to be exposed to FM and see it as a worthwhile career option. To meet this essential objective, FM departments are required in all medical schools. Studies indicate that, in the case of countries such as Bahrain and Saudi Arabia, there are substantially more medical graduates entering postgraduate training in FM, since they have departments of FM in their medical schools and teaching in FM at the undergraduate level. Medical education at the undergraduate level in most institutions in the EMR is substantially hospital-based, whereas it should be in combination with major exposure to community based activities.[1]

POSTGRADUATE TRAINING IN FAMILY MEDICINE

In the EMR, there is a general shortage of training programs that could provide trained human resources to work in FM departments. Strategies can be drawn from existing models in which training in FM has been successfully achieved in a short period of time. The Primafamed project involved 10 universities in eight Sub-Saharan countries in training family physicians in a span of two and a half years.[4] Primafamed has adopted a strategic approach, drawing on successful models from the developed world. Sudan is one EMR country to have already benefited from this model.

SHORT TRAINING FOR CAPACITY BUILDING OF GENERAL PRACTITIONERS

Several countries in the EMR claim to have short courses in FM for existing general practitioners (GPs), of up to a year in duration. A need for such short courses has been identified in FM. They are mostly run in the public sector and appear to fulfil short-term urgent needs. The private sector also needs to be involved in this endeavor. There are concerns whether family physicians are safe clinicians after going through these short courses. Curriculum, assessment, and accreditation issues need further strengthening. Accreditation of training programs can be either at a national level, such as by the Saudi Commission for Health Specialties in Saudi Arabia, or at the regional level, such as by the Arab Board of Family and Community Medicine. The World Health Organization needs to advocate for short courses in improving the capacities of GPs to ensure that the quality of practice of those undertaking these courses is guaranteed, and that such courses are allowed for a limited period of time until a sufficient number of postgraduate family medicine training programs have been established. Continuing Medical Education courses are also needed to raise the standards of practicing Family Doctors across the Region.[5]

Most EMR Member States have significant deficiencies in human resources for health, especially in Family Medicine. Member States need to make concerted efforts to introduce FM education and training at the undergraduate, postgraduate, and continuing professional development levels. Most countries in the EMR will need to go through a major transformation to redesign and strengthen their health-care systems from hospital-based systems, focusing on treating diseases, to community-based systems, with a focus on providing comprehensive basic, preventive, promotive, and curative health services to all their people.

REFERENCES

1. World Health Organization, Eastern Mediterranean Region Working Paper. Current Status of Family Medicine Education and Training in Eastern Mediterranean Region, 2014.
2. Kidd M. The Contribution of Family Medicine to Improving Health Systems. A Guidebook from the World Organization of Family Doctors (2nd edition), 2013. New York: Radcliffe Publishing London.
3. Alnasir FAL. Family medicine in the Arab world? Is it a luxury? *Journal of the Bahrain Medical Society*, 2009; 21(1): 191–192.
4. Flinkenflögel M, Essuman A, Patrick Chege P, Ayankogbe O, and Maeseneer JD. Family medicine training in sub-Saharan Africa: South-South cooperation in the Primafamed project as strategy for development. *Family Practice*, 2014; 31(4): 427–436.
5. Anwar H, Batty H. Continuing medical education strategy for primary health care physicians in Oman: lessons to be learnt. *Oman Medical Journal*, 2007; 22(3): 33–35.

CHAPTER 9

Leveraging technology to transition general practitioners to the family practice model of care

Ghassan Hamadeh, Mona Osman, and Hossein Hamam

The World Health Organization (WHO) Regional Office for the Eastern Mediterranean (EMRO) has adopted the concept of family practice for achieving Universal Health Coverage.[1] We describe here the use of eLearning tools for the transition of experienced general practitioners (GP) to the family practice model of care.

Family practice is characterized by eight attributes, namely the provision of general, first contact, continuous, comprehensive, coordinated, and collaborative care with an orientation towards the family and the community.[2] A curriculum for training GPs/family physicians is expected to facilitate the acquisition of the core competencies defined by the World Organization of Family Doctors: primary care management, person-centred care, problem-solving skills, comprehensive approach, community-orientation, and holistic approach.[3]

The main challenge facing the implementation of family practice in the Eastern Mediterranean Region is the limited number of available family medicine training programs and practicing family physicians.[4] Although expanding the number of training programs is the preferred approach to this challenge, upgrading the skills of GPs in the family practice model through bridging professional development programs is an alternative.[4] Grandfathering or bridging programs leading to diplomas or certificates have been adopted by numerous countries.

Technological advances have revolutionized traditional methods of teaching by making it possible for educators to have virtual classrooms available to a larger audience according to the latter's time and location convenience. This mode of learning is ideal for working professionals. The exclusive use of online training is not validated, especially in the health sectors.[5] This may be why most universities continue the use of "blended learning", which merges web-based training with face-to-face activities.

The Department of Family Medicine at the American University of Beirut Medical Center was approached by WHO-EMRO to develop an "Advanced General Practice" update course. The course targets GPs who have not received any vocational or postgraduate training prior to entering practice. It complements the experience these practitioners have acquired in their career and hopes to re-focus them on the main components of the family practice model.

The course spans over a period of 24 weeks and uses the Moodle Learning Management System in a blended format. This format is intended to accommodate the work schedule of the GPs, and it allows continuous online interaction between the tutors and trainees.

The course includes an orientation session, four teaching blocks (including web-based presentations, online discussions, on-the-job training sessions and live reviews), and an exam period. The evaluation of trainees is based on formative and summative assessments. A course director and an information technology specialist are needed for the proper implementation of the course.

The course was first implemented in 2017 with 16 GPs working with the United Nations Relief and Works Agency in Lebanon. GPs were divided into three groups with a tutor assigned to each group. Tutors followed-up with the trainees on a weekly basis online and conducted on-the-job training twice per block. GPs were expected to complete web-based presentations and online quizzes weekly, one assignment per block, and attend one live review session per block. At the conclusion of the four-block course, GPs were evaluated through a written final exam and an Objective Structure Clinical Examination. The course implementation was smooth and the feedback from GPs revealed great satisfaction with the content and modality of training.

Technology is a viable method to transition GPs into the family practice model of care. This course is offered as a university-based structured continuous professional development in general practice. Moving forward, and to accelerate the transition to the family practice model across the region, a full bridging programme should be adopted by specialty licensing bodies until a satisfactory number of full-fledged residency training programs has been established.

REFERENCES

1. EMRO. Conceptual and strategic approach to family practice: Towards universal health coverage through family practice in the Eastern Mediterranean Region. 2014; Available from: http://applications.emro.who.int/dsaf/EMROPUB_2014_EN_1783.pdf [Accessed 17 November 2017].
2. Kidd, M.R. *The Contribution of Family Medicine to Improving Health Systems: A guidebook from the World Organization of Family Doctors* (2nd edition), 2013. London, New York: Radcliffe Pub. xxvii, 293 p.
3. WONCA. The European Definition of General Practice/Family Medicine. 2011 [Accessed 17 November 2017].
4. EMRO. *Scaling up family practice: Progressing towards universal health coverage.* Regional Committee for the Eastern Mediterranean - Technical Papers 2016; EM/RC63/Tech.Disc.1 Rev.1 [Accessed 17 November 2017].
5. McCutcheon, K. et al., A systematic review evaluating the impact of online or blended learning vs. face-to-face learning of clinical skills in undergraduate nurse education. *Journal of Advanced Nursing,* 2015, 71(2): 255–270.

CHAPTER 10

Measuring the quality of primary health care: a regional initiative in the Eastern Mediterranean Region

Mondher Letaief, Lisa Hirschhorn,
Aziz Sheikh, and Sameen Siddiqi

To strengthen the measurement of primary health care (PHC) to drive change, the World Health Organization (WHO) Regional Office for the Eastern Mediterranean Region (EMRO) embarked on a process to identify and test a core set of indicators to improve the quality of health-care delivery through better measurement to drive improvement. The process included a strategic series of activities including literature review, expert input, pilot testing, regional conferences for sharing information, and iteration of a set of core measures.

The methodology of the process involved a series of steps including the creation of a framework, which involved the continuum of health care and Donabedian's classic framework.[1] This was then overlaid with the six core dimensions of quality.[2] Quality of Care Indicators were then selected, considering the three critical characteristics of any indicator: importance, validity, and feasibility. This selection process included Initial Indicator Selection through a rapid scoping review of the existing literature, using the search terms "quality of care", "indicators", and "measures", and the development of a candidate indicator matrix. The review of the literature was supplemented by input from experts in the area of quality of care and primary care from across the Eastern Mediterranean Region (EMR). This was followed by an eDelphi Process involving 27 experts external to and from the region to review the candidate indicators[3,] and then Small-Scale Pilot Testing was carried out in three PHC facilities in Egypt and two PHC centres of the United Nations Relief and Works Agency for Palestine Refugees (UNRWA) in Jordan. This work led to refining the set of priority indicators, as well as suggested modifications on operational definitions. A final list of 34 indicators[4], covering six domains of quality (access, equity, safety, efficiency, effectiveness, and patient-centredness), with each domain split into three subcategories (structure, process, and outcomes), was developed for broader testing. A toolkit was developed to further test the feasibility of indicator measurement, data availability, and challenges and gaps. The measurement of the identified indicator set using the toolkit was implemented through a five-step process in 10 facilities in each of four countries (Iran, Jordan, Oman, Tunisia) and through facilities run by UNRWA.

The results from testing in the four countries and with UNRWA showed wide variability between and within countries on both data availability and the results. In terms of patient-centredness, only two countries had enough data, with rates of 44% and 64%, while 53% and 77% in those same countries were aware of patients' rights and responsibilities.

While immunization rates for children under 23 months were generally high (from 82% to 100%), influenza vaccination was much lower. Percentage of registered hypertension patients with BP <140/90 at the last two follow- up visits was from 32% to 73%, and percentage of registered diabetic patients with HbA1C under 7% ranged from 16% to 56%. The percentage of diabetes mellitus patients who had had fundus eye examination during the last 12 months, or the percentage of registered NCD patients with blood pressure recorded twice at last follow-up visit, were on average 45% and 40% respectively.

Key conclusions from this research included the need to adapt the indicators for adoption into existing country contexts, the recognition of current challenges to the full measurement of the core indicators, and that planned measurement work needed to include capacity building for data collection and use, including supervision.

Some countries have shown commitment in PHC quality measurement: Iran has established a national committee which is working on the next steps; Oman has started with field implementation of the indicators; Sudan has adapted the indicators, trained focal points from its states, and added some indicators to reflect country priorities and which can be integrated with the National Quality Policy and Strategy to ensure they are included in the national priorities for health.

The Regional Committee of the EMR has since approved a resolution on adopting quality indicators for improving the quality of care at the primary care level.[5]

Measurement of quality is a critical step towards identifying areas for strengthening, as well as needed strategies and interventions. This needs to occur within and across countries for local action and regional benchmarking.[6] This work has resulted in a number of findings and recommendations for work within WHO EMRO and beyond, including demonstrating the feasibility of creating a regional indicator set, the importance of stakeholder engagement, the need to build on existing work and measures but allowing local adaptation, the need to measure what matters, and the need to ensure people-centredness in the indicators developed.

There were a number of challenges recognized which some of the countries have already begun to address. Recommendations for future work include the need to include all sectors in national quality measurement work, the need to address measuring quality in the context of conflict, the need to measure aspirational goals and ensure flexibility to cover priorities across a diverse set of health systems, and the need to continue work to adapt or develop better tools.

REFERENCES

1. Donabedian A. The quality of care. How can it be assessed? *JAMA*. 1988;260(12):1743–1748.
2. Institute of Medicine (US) Committee on Quality of Health Care in America. *Crossing the Quality Chasm: A New Health System for the 21st Century.* Washington (DC): National Academies Press (US); 2001. Available from: http://www.ncbi.nlm.nih.gov/books/NBK222274/ [Accessed 20 March 2017].
3. Refinement of indicators and criteria in a quality tool for assessing quality in primary care in Canada: a Delphi Panel study. Available from: https://pdfs.semanticscholar.org/3b92/ab32d4c42ea92e8613f467 02707ae2336fd8.pdf [Accessed 2/3/2017].
4. Salah H and Kidd M. Family Practice in the Eastern Mediterranean Region: Universal Health Coverage and Quality Primary Care. Available from: https://www.amazon.com/Family-Practice-Eastern-Mediterranean-SPECIAL-ebook/dp/B07K4T8TFR [Accessed 19/01/2019].
5. WHO EMRO. Scaling up family practice: progressing towards universal health coverage. Available from: http://applications.emro.who.int/docs/RC63_ Resolutions_2016_R2_19197_EN.pdf
6. WHO. Quality of care: measuring a neglected driver of improved health. Available from: http://www.who.int/bulletin/volumes/95/6/16-180190/en/ [Accessed 9/02/2017].

CHAPTER 11

The challenge of providing Primary Health Care services in crisis countries in the Eastern Mediterranean Region

Xavier Mòdol

The World Health Organization (WHO) Eastern Mediterranean Region (EMR) presently is the arena of the world's major conflicts and over one-third of its member countries have been in permanent conflict for the last five years or more.

The health impact of conflict includes increased morbidity and mortality as a consequence of violence.[1] Wars and conflict have increasingly become protracted, targeting civilians as well as socio-economic infrastructure, and creating mass population displacement that often settle in urban settings, among the regular dwellers rather than in refugee/IDP (Internally Displaced People) camps.[2] Long periods of low-intensity conflict tend to produce fewer violent deaths but more long-term health effects, with increased prevalence of mental health conditions, tuberculosis, and even non-communicable diseases. A worrisome finding is the re-emergence of communicable diseases, of which the region had been free for more than one decade, such as poliomyelitis (Syria, Iraq) and diphtheria (Yemen), and which reflects the collapse of routine immunization systems.[3] System collapse also is at the roots of the occurrence in Yemen of a cholera epidemic of unprecedented dimensions.

Conflict may limit access to health services by reducing the system's capacity through different mechanisms, including the actual destruction of the health facility, the disruption of supply chains or the displacement of skilled health workers. Health facilities and personnel are becoming targets in increasingly sickening conflicts.[4]

Primary health care (PHC) service organization is influenced, among others, by the phase of the conflict, from open war to peace building, or the variety of different authorities that administer a territory previously unified. Open conflict is characterized by the presence of humanitarian actors – usually non-governmental organizations (NGOs), and the setting up of coping delivery models, such as the so-called "field hospitals" in the Syrian conflict. Support is provided to individual facilities rather than systems and the role of the government is diminished. Mass displacement means that a large part of PHC may be delivered outside the country.

Peace building and stabilization may bring changes in the delivery model, such as the contracting out to NGO providers in Afghanistan, Somalia or Darfur, or the inclusion of Mental Health or non-communicable disease (NCD) management in service packages provided.

Essential Packages of Health Services (EPHS) are promoted as an effective, efficient and standardized way of scaling up service delivery, often as a part of a sector reform process. EPHS may be specific to humanitarian contexts, such as the Sphere project and the Minimum Initial Service Package (MISP). Although most EMR countries in conflict have developed their EPHS, there is little evidence of implementation, with Afghanistan as the main exception.

Crisis situations coincide with reduced fiscal space of the involved government, resulting in reduced government health expenditure. The main alternatives are external resources and out-of-pocket (OOP) expenditure. The Global Health Expenditure Database gives levels of OOP of 76% of total health expenditure in Yemen and Sudan, 64% in Afghanistan, and 54% in Syria, compared to 20% in Jordan, 35% in Tunisia, and 15% in Saudi Arabia. Donor funding has proven instrumental in infrastructure/reconstruction projects or on the financing of health reform interventions, often responding to an external agenda.

Delivering the combination of services that comprise PHC requires that the right combination of skills operates in the right locations. Country health systems should ensure proper supply, adequate distribution and performance-informed management of staff for these basic teams to be able to perform their duties. Some of the factors influencing the performance of health care workers, such as knowledge and skills, motivation, availability of updated clinical guidelines, availability of equipment, medicines and supplies, and supportive evaluation, are not easy to access and enforce, particularly in challenging contexts. Training capacity, and particularly the standards of quality of training, are among the first casualties in a conflict situation. Attrition of cadres of health care workers, and even migration to safer contexts, is high during the first phases of the crisis, but also substantial is their replacement by foreign and volunteer humanitarian workers.[5] Adequate distribution of the health care workforce is hindered by insecurity, low salaries and lack of appealing retention packages.

The adoption by many countries of the Family Practice (FP) approach has linked this strategy to the presence of a specialized health care worker, the Family Medicine (FM) specialist. This presents the double challenge of developing a training and certification package that can be appealing to some of the best physicians in the country, and finding a solution for the many doctors who will not achieve that certification. There are several FM programmes in EMR countries, however there has been a reduced output of certified specialists.[6]

In countries where access to basic health services is not guaranteed by formal delivery systems, new cadres may be created, recruited and trained to operate in the remotest, most insecure locations. In Afghanistan, training and recruitment of Community Midwives[7] has been accelerated to increase skilled deliveries in remote areas where no urban-trained professional would accept a position. Community Health Workers (CHWs) have been used as a replacement for the provision of at least some PHC components.

Each crisis requires a tailored approach to delivering PHC. Time and again, resilient health systems bounce back to provide the closest they can to a standard range of PHC services. Having a structured vision for the future may help navigate the stormy waters of the present, but appropriate adjustment should happen almost on a daily basis.

REFERENCES

1. C. Murray, G. King, A. Lopez, N. Tomijima and E. Krug. Armed conflict as a public health problem. *British Medical Journal,* 2002; 324: 346–9.
2. P. Spiegel, F. Checchi, S. Colombo and E. Paik. Health-care needs of people affected by conflict: future trends and changing frameworks. *Lancet,* 2010; 375: 341–45.
3. R. Raslan, S. El Sayegh, S. Chams, N. Chams, A. Leone and I. Hussein. Re-emerging Vaccine-Preventable Diseases in War-Affected Peoples of the Eastern Mediterranean Region—An Update. *Frontiers in Public Health,* 2017; 5.
4. S. Colombo and E. Pavignani. Recurrent failings of medical humanitarianism: intractable, ignored, or just exaggerated? *Lancet (online),* 2017.
5. E. Pavignani. Human Resources for Health Under Stress in the Eastern Mediterranean Region. World Health Organization, 2017.
6. A. Abyad, A. Al-Baho, I. Unluoglu, M. Tarawneh and T. Al Hilfy. Development of Family Medicine in the Middle East. *Family Medicine,* 2007; 39 (10): 736–41.
7. X. Mòdol. Afghanistan Joint Health Sector Review and Strategic Plan Implementation Assessment. European Union, Ministry of Public Health of Afghanistan, Kabul, 2015.

CHAPTER 12

Public–private partnerships: The Mazandaran experience on contracting with private family physicians, Islamic Republic of Iran

Mohsen A'arabi, Mohsen Asadi-Lari, and Ghasem Janbabaei

Mazandaran province is located in northern Iran on the coast of the Caspian Sea with a population of 3,283,582 people (1,756,456 are living in urban areas).

The Rural Family Medicine Program began in the rural areas of Mazandaran province in 2005, by basing rural family physicians and midwives in rural health centres responsible for people's health supporting the Behvarzes, community health workers based in village health houses and with responsibility for providing health service packages to all people. The coverage of this program is complete. A referral system is in place between each village health house and its rural health centre. Family physician and midwife salaries are calculated on a per capita basis.

In contrast, the provision of services was not integrated in urban health facilities. Therefore, the need for a family physician-based approach for service delivery for urban areas, as well as in rural areas, was considered by policymakers and members of Parliament.[1] A steering committee, executive committee, and a monitoring and evaluation committee, were established at the provincial level with involvement of the main stakeholders.

Private sector physicians interested in working as urban family physicians, without any dual practice, apply to the District Health Center. They are also obligated to employ a midwife/nurse to work in their office. To sign a contract with insurance organizations, the application is examined by both district and provincial levels of the health network. Insurance organizations are responsible for direct payments to family physicians after monthly approvals of their service provision. Over the past five years, more than 78% of 637 family physicians applying in Mazandaran have had contracts with insurance agencies for over three years.[2]

The population covered by each full-time family physician post is 2500 people. Eight hours of service delivery per day is provided to ensure better access of people to services. In a study of 1768 randomly selected families within the Mazandaran province, the average time required to reach the family physician was reported as 16.3 minutes on foot, or 5.6 minutes by car.

Using the private sector's capacity to cover the population was one of the best available solutions, as there was no need for governmental investment in the construction and equipping of new offices, or the employment of extra human resources. At the start of the contract, physicians need to have a suitable physical space, with an area of at least 40 m², and the equipment required on the standard list. The family physician should also nominate a locum physician in case of absence, to ensure continuity of care. For part-time family physicians, a locum physician for both morning and afternoon shifts is required. Monitoring of the family physician's performance is carried out by other family physicians and health experts from the comprehensive health centre in the family physician's area. Additional monitoring visits are carried out by the insurance organizations and the city health centre. Results of this monitoring system are used for payments of 20% of the per-capita every three months. First-level health service packages are provided by the Ministry of Health and Medical Education, based on the age groups of the covered population, and notified to all family physicians. These age groups include neonates, children, adolescents, youth, middle-aged, elderly, and pregnant and lactating mothers.

In a study of 96 urban family physicians, the overall satisfaction of physicians involved in the program was 3.37 out of 5. In contrast, a survey of 888 people in 2016, showed 23.8% had changed their family physician once and 2.8% had changed their physician twice or more during the past 12 months. With regard to satisfaction with the services provided, 62.8% were satisfied and 37.2% were dissatisfied.

During the implementation of this program, several problems came to light, including a lack of equivalent funds provided by insurance organizations; insufficient competencies among family physicians in providing health promotion services and primary prevention; unwillingness of specialists to play their role and provide advice and feedback to family physicians; delays in monthly per-capita payments to family physicians; low awareness and cultural acceptance of family physician services among the population; and delay in access to efficient electronic health records.

After nearly five years of experience since the implementation of the urban family physician program in Mazandaran province, the following initiatives are being developed in order to improve performance: a complete performance-based payment system, encouraging family physicians to work in groups instead of solo, raising the competencies of family physicians and health experts through education, using team-based training models for family physician team education, advocacy for access to sustainable financial resources and regular payments and reform in the payment systems for specialist and sub-specialist physicians.

REFERENCES

1. Aarabi M, Oveis G, Alaei O. *Urban Family Physician in Mazandaran Province.* Sary, Mazandaran (Iran): Mazandaran University of Medical Sciences and Health Services, Deputy of Public Health; 2017. Report No. 3.
2. Nasrollahpour Shirvani SD, Kabir MJ, Ashrafian Amiri H, Rabiei SM, Keshavarzi A, Farzin K. *Experience of Implementing the Program of the Urban Family Physician in Iran.* 1st edition. Tehran: Iran Health Organization, 2017: 93.

CHAPTER 13

Afghanistan

Bashir Noormal, Najibullah Safi, and Shafiqullah Hemat

Total number of primary health-care (PHC) facilities	2067
Number of general practitioners working in public PHC facilities	2941
Number of certified family physicians working in PHC facilities	70
Average number of family physician graduates/year	8
Number of medical schools	37 (public 9, private 28)
Number of family medicine departments in medical schools	2

INTRODUCTION

The Afghanistan Health System has the Basic Package of Health Services (BPHS) and the Essential Package of Hospital Services (EPHS). The BPHS provides primary care and preventive services, whereas the EPHS consists of hospital-level services. District hospitals have elements of both categories of services. Besides these two packages, there is another group of hospitals called speciality/national hospitals, which are referral centres for tertiary medical care.[1]

BPHS and EPHS delivery is funded and contracted through the Government of Islamic Republic Afghanistan (GoIRA) health systems and accompanied by technical assistance to the Ministry of

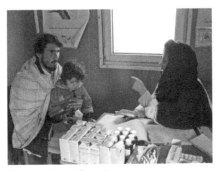

Pharmacist with patient

Public Health (MoPH) by multiple development partners. The GoIRA directs the delivery of health services, but delivery itself is accomplished largely by non-governmental organizations. Funding for the public health system comes almost exclusively from external resources. Over time, the GoIRA will gradually need to become the principal provider of funds to the health sector. Donors will continue to fund delivery of the BPHS and EPHS across all 34 provinces of the country to year 2021.

KEY CHALLENGES

Afghanistan faces the serious challenges of a fragile political environment, continued threats from insurgencies and local power holders, economic downturn, diminishing aid flows, widespread corruption, and regional relationships that continue to exacerbate conflict. These complex factors and associated dynamics have had significant adverse impacts on state effectiveness and all aspects of Afghanistan's development, including in the health sector. Afghanistan has the highest total fertility rate in Asia, at 5.3 children born/woman; its population is now growing by almost 1 million people annually.[3,4] In general, Afghanistan's "hard infrastructure", including roads and reliable supplies of water and power, is inadequate to support expanded and effective health service delivery and access. The health status of maternal, newborn, and child health is among the worst in the world. Malnutrition is a serious problem; according to a recent report by UNICEF, 59% of children suffer from childhood stunting, making it the worst in the world. Health expenditures in the country are tilted towards out-of-pocket spending by families which accounts for 74% of all spending.

WAY FORWARD

The MoPH has seven strategic directions: [1] Healthy public policy/health in all policies, [2] Supportive environment, [3] Community actions, [4] Develop Personal Skills, [5] Reorient health services, [6] Capacity Building, [7] Coordination and partnership.

The MoPH has 10 operating principles: [1] Country-owned and country-led development, [2] Good governance, including effective transparency and accountability,[1] [3] The right to health for all, especially women, children, and members of vulnerable groups, [4] Gender balance, [5] Leverage strengths through internal and external partnerships and coordination, [6] Effective community involvement and participation, [7] Culture of evidence-based planning, decision making, results orientation, and results-based management, [8] The promotion of "systems thinking" at all levels, [9] A culture of togetherness and team and cross-functional work, [10] Emphasis on health promotion and prevention.[2]

Improved access and expansion of coverage has led to some impressive results. The infant mortality ratio has declined from 66 deaths per 1000 live births in 2005, to 45 in 2017. During the same period, neonatal mortality has dropped from 31 to 22, under-five mortality from 87 to 55 per 1000 live births, and skilled birth attendance has increased from 14% in 2003, to more than 50% in 2017.[4] The decline in the maternal mortality rate also has been dramatic, falling from 1600 to 396 per 100,000 live births.[3] There has also been a significant increase in the coverage of key maternal and child health service indicators; antenatal coverage increased from 16% to 59%, the contraceptive prevalence rate rose from 10% to 23%, institutional deliveries from under 15% to 48%, and DPT3/Penta 3 coverage for children of ages 0 to 23 months increased from 30% to 58%.[4]

REFERENCES

1. Essential Package of Health Services for Afghanistan, 2005.
2. Ministry of Public Health. *Afghanistan Health Indicators Fact Sheet.* 2014. Available from: http://mop h.gov.af/Content/Media/Documents/AfghanistanHealthIndicatorsFactsheetFeb201461220141026165155 3325325.pdf [Accessed 31 January 2018].
3. Central Statistics Organization (CSO), Ministry of Public Health (MoPH), and ICF. *Afghanistan Demographic and Health Survey 2015.* Kabul, Afghanistan, and Rockville, Maryland, USA. 2017.
4. Central Statistics Organization. *National Risk and Vulnerability Assessment 2011–12. Afghanistan Living Condition Survey.* Kabul, CSO. 2012.

CHAPTER 14

Bahrain

Faisal Abdullatif Alnasir and Adel Al-Sayyad

Total number of PHC facilities	28
Number of general practitioners working in public PHC facilities	98
Number of certified family physicians working in PHC facilities	228
Average number of family physician graduates/year	22
Number of medical schools	2
Number of family medicine departments	1

INTRODUCTION

Bahrain fulfilled the United Nation's Millennium Development Goals in the health sector five years before the agreed schedule of 2015.[1] The life expectancy rate in the Kingdom had significantly increased, reaching 77.2 years in 2015, compared to 73.4 years in 2000.[2] This has led to an increase in the population of elderly people who have more health-care needs.[3]

Most of the essential facilities and services, including family medicine, are available within the nation's PHC centers. In each specific health centre, only people within its geographical distribution are registered and they are not permitted to consult other health centers without a referral. The curative and preventive services that are provided by the centers are under the direct supervision of family physicians. More often, each family is assigned to a specific doctor (i.e. their own family physician).

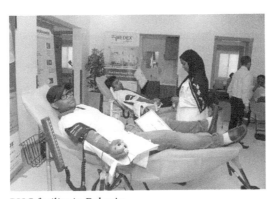

PHC facility in Bahrain

Recently electronic medical records (I-Seha) were introduced and within I-Seha the patient's information is saved to a server and can be shared, with permission, by different sections of the health system such as secondary care, tertiary care, and other health facilities.

The primary health-care service is provided free of charge for Bahrainis and for a fee for expatriates if they are not insured. Within PHC there is a good referral system to secondary care, should the patient need further investigation, treatment, or a second opinion. Later all the information is fed back to the referring doctor.

The family medicine programme started in 1979, which was a milestone in health sector improvement. All credit goes to the courageous decision that was taken by a politician, the former Minister of Health, Dr Ali Fakhroo, who was a strong believer and advocate for family medicine and who had a vision for the health of the nation which proved to be the right one for the country.

KEY CHALLENGES

Although Bahrain was the first country in the Gulf region to start its residency programme in family medicine, and to establish primary health-care services for its population, it faces many challenges that may prevent it from applying a full-fledged family medicine service. One of the most important obstacles is the shortage of family doctors produced to date, which is far less than is needed. The country with its present population requires 696 well-trained family doctors, while the available workforce is nearly half of that, making a family doctor to population ratio of 1 to 3580 which is far less than optimal. The second serious challenge, which is also related to the shortage of family physicians, is that the fully qualified family doctors are overloaded with patients during their day to day practice giving them less time to implement ideal family medicine practice.

WAY FORWARD

To overcome those challenges, a firm strategy must be adopted by policy makers that entails the following:

- The government should have a clear strategy of considering family medicine and primary health care as the foundation of the health system in the country.
- There should be an increase in the health-care budget which is allocated to primary health care services, compared to the budget allocated to secondary and tertiary care services.
- Moreover, a brave decision ought to be taken to increase the number of specialized family physicians by increasing the number of residency programmes to more than one, and by increasing the intake capacity of the existing programme to more than thirty doctors per year. The current production rate of 16 new family doctors graduating each year means it will take at least 22 years to produce the number of family physicians the country needs.

REFERENCES

1. Bahrain Health Care. http://www.bahrain.com/en/bi/key-investment-sectors/Pages/Healthcare.aspx#.WfrU Aztx3cs [Accessed 22 September 2018].
2. Ministry of Health statistics 2015. https://www.moh.gov.bh/Content/Files/Publications/statistics/HS2015/hs2015_e.htm [Accessed 22 September 2018].
3. Alnasir Faisal "Ageing and Pattern of Population Changes in the Developing Countries". *The Middle East Journal of Age & Aging.* 2015: 12:2; 26–32.

CHAPTER 15

Djibouti

Abdoulaye Konate

Total number of primary health-care facilities	71
Number of general practitioners working in public primary health-care institutions	51
Number of certified family doctors working in primary health-care institutions	0
Average number of family medicine graduates per year	0
Number of medical schools	1
Number of family medicine departments	0

INTRODUCTION

The government has stepped up efforts to increase the number of primary health-care facilities, especially health posts which rose from 22 in 2004 to 38 in 2016, a 73% increase. During the same period, the number of health centres rose from 8 to 15, an increase of 88%. In addition to the semi-public sector, there are 10 primary health-care facilities. Family practice and family medicine have not been adopted yet for implementation in Djibouti. With the aim of strengthening the preventive sector, the government has set up the Djibouti National Institute of Public Health, facilities for priority health areas such as maternal and child health, immunization, malaria, TB, and human immunodeficiency virus (HIV), in addition to providing curative care. All these government initiatives have helped to improve the PHC situation in Djibouti, although further efforts need to be made to reduce the burden of disease on the population.

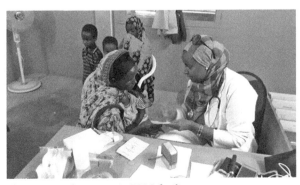

Physician with patient in PHC facility

Maternal and child health has seen an improvement, with the number of maternal deaths per 100,000 live births decreasing from 740 in 1996, to 383 in 2012, a reduction of almost 50%. Between 2002 and 2012, infant and child mortality fell from 131 to 68 per 1000 live births, infant mortality fell from 108 to 68 per 1000 live births, and neonatal mortality fell from 45 to 36 per 1000 live births.[1] The prevalence of TB in 2014 was 906 cases per 100,000 inhabitants. Incidence has been decreasing, with 378 new cases per 100,000 inhabitants in 2015, down from 619 new cases in 2013. Despite this downward trend, Djibouti still has one of the highest rates of TB in the world. The integration of basic health services has been one of the priorities of Djibouti's government for many years.[2]

The country's health map, created in 2006, set out a Minimum Package of integrated services. There is a referral and counter-referral system between the different levels of the health pyramid. This system makes direct admissions for patients easier, and treatment is free of charge. For adults, transfers and referrals are not as well-organized and are chargeable. In line with the PHC strategy, the health system has been making essential generic medicines available since 2003, updated in 2016. Human resources for health have seen a substantial increase. In 2016, there were 1.06 general practitioners per 10,000 inhabitants, and 8.18 paramedical staff per 10,000 inhabitants.[3] The health-care workforce rose from 1664 in 2008, to 3381 in 2017, an increase of more than 100%.

KEY CHALLENGES

According to the results of the 2015 Service Availability and Readiness Assessment, the availability index of health infrastructures on a national level is 38.9%. In fact, two-thirds of the country's regions have not reached the national average. No studies have been performed to illustrate the prevalence, incidence, and patterns of Non-communicable diseases (NCDs). NCDs are responsible for 40% of hospital admissions and one-third of hospital deaths at Hôpital Général Peltier in Djibouti City. Djibouti still does not have a quality and accreditation programme for its health services. For most diseases, there are no protocols harmonized on a national level. Integration efforts need to be made in PHC, and screening, treatment, and monitoring of NCDs. 43% of under-five deaths in Djibouti are linked to malnutrition. In terms of health financing, challenges lie in the need to increase the budget allocated to health care from the general budget, attracting funding from external sources, and expanding the scope for Universal Health Insurance.

WAY FORWARD

To improve the quality of primary health care services, the following actions are needed: [1] Developing community health activities, [2] Adapting health care to meet patients' needs, [3] Extending a high-quality approach to hospitals and specialized centres, [4] Ensuring continuity of care between the different levels, from the community up, [5] Improving preparedness of the health system to manage migration flows and humanitarian crises, [6] Increasing health-care access for rural and cut-off populations, [6] Developing an integrated strategy for health promotion, [7] Updating the minimum package of activities, with a focus on integrating services, particularly for NCDs, [8] Developing partnerships and contractual relationships, [9] Drawing up a roadmap for comprehensively reforming the health information system, [10] Drawing up a strategic development plan for human resources.

REFERENCES

1. Survey final report, Pan Arab Project for Family Health (PAPFAM), Djibouti. 2012.
2. National Health Statistics, Djibouti. 2016.
3. Annual Report of the Financial and Human Resources Department, Djibouti. 2017.

CHAPTER 16

Egypt

Omaima El-Gibaly, Magdy Bakr, Mona Hafez Mahmoud El Naka, Taghreed Mohamed Farahat, and Nagwa Nashat Hegazy

Total number of PHC facilities	5,391
Number of general practitioners working in public PHC facilities	14,973
Number of certified family physicians working in PHC facilities	256
Average number of family physician graduates/year	180
Number of medical schools	29
Number of family medicine departments	8

INTRODUCTION

Egypt's Family Practice (FP) was established in 1999 as one of Egypt's health sector reform programme strategies. It was structured as an integrated approach to providing basic health services and was commonly called the "Family Health Model" (FHM).[1] As per its original design, the model has been an integrated approach to provide geographical coverage to families with basic services, including both health and population interventions. Each family physician, supported by a multidisciplinary health team, serves a roster of families within the catchment area of the health facility ranging between 5000 and 10,000 households.

The development of a basic service package to be provided to all Egypt's population was one of the key components of Egypt's Health Sector Reform Programme initiated in 1997 – and was named the "Basic Benefits Package (BBP)".

Improving the quality of services was a prime goal of Egypt's Health Sector Reform Programme. As part of the programme strategies, a "Quality Improvement Directorate" was established by "Ministerial Decree" (number 272 for the year 1998). The quality directorate developed a comprehensive programme to improve quality through designing and implementing an accreditation system. In July 2007, the Egyptian accreditation standards for hospitals, ambulatory care, and PHC was accredited by the International Society for Quality in Health-care (ISQua) making Egypt the first country in the region to attain this certificate[2].

Implementation and development of the FHM in Egypt is considered a strong contribution to UHC as it entails providing integrated and quality services to the entire population and considers

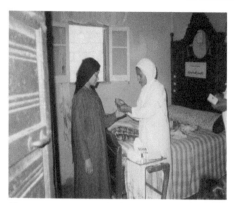

Community outreach through FHM

their psychosocial well-being along with well-defined social protection mechanisms where the health care needs of the poor and members of vulnerable populations are covered by the state[3].

KEY CHALLENGES

- As part of fragmentation of the whole health system, there is fragmentation in institutional and regulatory frameworks.
- One of the major challenges identified is ensuring sufficient, well-educated, trained, adequately paid and motivated health teams in family health facilities.
- There are recurrent shortages of medicines to support the service package.
- Information management suffers from manual records, fragmentation, duplication, and lagging automation, as well as weak information sharing and use.
- A dysfunctional referral system with no institutional arrangements.
- Community participation is rather "theoretical".

WAY FORWARD

- Institutional and regulatory arrangements: Revise, update, and standardize the FHM's institutional, regulatory, and financial frameworks.
- Resolve or rectify issues related to the mandatory service by medical graduates (called "takleef").
- Rationalize medical records and registration, avoiding duplication and multiple streaming.
- Develop a well-balanced service package through systematic analysis of burden of disease and costing studies.
- Develop and implement solid institutional arrangements to mandate referral of clearly identified services.
- Implement strategic purchasing of family health services through contracts with appropriate provider payment mechanisms as an efficient way of improving provider performance.
- Enhance the role of the community through strengthening community-based initiatives.

REFERENCES

1. Lie DA, Boker JR, Lenahan PM, Dow E, Scherger, JE. An international physician education program to support the recent introduction of family medicine in Egypt. *Family Medicine,* 2004; 36(10): 739–746.
2. Roadmap to achieve social justice in health care in Egypt. *World Bank.* 2015.
3. Devi S. Universal health coverage law approved in Egypt. *Lancet,* 2018; 391(10117): 194. Available from: https://www.thelancet.com/journals/lancet/article/PIIS0140–6736(18)30091–6/fulltext [Accessed 22 September 2018].

CHAPTER 17

Islamic Republic of Iran

Mohammadreza Rahbar, Alireza Raeisi, Mohsen Asadi-Lari, and Hasti Sanaei-Shoar

Total number of PHC facilities	27,173
Number of general practitioners working in public PHC facilities	9,500
Number of universities of medical sciences (public)	66
Number of medical schools	85
Number of general practitioners with MFM (Master of Family Medicine 2-year course)	1,000
Number of family medicine specialists	86
Number of family medicine residents	174

INTRODUCTION

Different plans and projects during a four-decade period have shaped the current Primary health care (PHC) network and its movement towards family practice and Universal Health Coverage (UHC). Three phases can be defined for the formation of the current health network.

The first phase involved developing the PHC network. The basic policies for this stage were, priority of prevention over treatment, priority of remote and underprivileged rural areas over urban areas, and finally priority of out-patient over in-patient services. The West Azerbaijan project, which started in 1971, was one of the most significant measures that led to the start of this phase.[1] The large scale establishment of the PHC network started from 1984 and, over a ten-year period, 90% of the rural population was covered with PHC services.[2] In 2019, over 98% of the rural population is covered by PHC services via 17,884 Health Houses (HHs) as the first level of delivering services and 2644 Rural Health Centres (HCs) as the second level of care. Almost the same services are delivered to urban communities, with 4111 Health Posts (HPs) as the first level and 2534 Urban Health Centres (HCs) as the second level. The Master Plan defines where the facilities should be located.[3] The HH are run by community health workers (behvarz). They are multipotential community health workers (CHWs) who pass a task-oriented training course.[4] The HPs are staffed by different health-care experts. Rural and Urban HCs are staffed by general practitioners, health technicians, and administrative personnel.[5]

The second phase involved developing Family Practice (FP) in rural areas and in cities with populations under 20,000. This phase started with a parliamentary decision, made in 2005, for legislation for Family Practice. The Health Insurance Organisation was obliged to issue health insurance cards for all residents of rural areas and urban communities with a population under 20,000. These services were to be implemented in the framework of the family practice and referral system.[6] The health

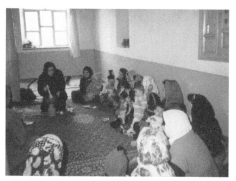

A behvarz training mothers to cook food for
their children

teams, with new members, started delivering new services in the HCs which were then called Centres
of Comprehensive Health Services (CCHS)[7]. Various programmes have been developed to enhance
the ability of family physicians, as well as members of the health team, including revising the educational syllabus of health staff, a Master of Family Medicine (MFM) Virtual Modular Course[8], and a
family medicine specialty programme.

The third phase was developing Family Practice in cities with populations of more than 20,000
people. The target population of this phase of the programme includes populations living in urban
areas, including the marginal populations around cities, and cities with more than 20,000 people. The
programme aims to implement UHC all over the country. This programme is based on public-private
partnerships (PPP), and devolution of services to the nongovernmental sector.

CHALLENGES

Demographic transition, with an increase in the elderly population with a higher burden of NCDs,
and increasing health expenses and limitation of resources, is the main challenge for the Iranian
health system. Increased marginalization, and lack of adequate health coverage in these areas, is the
second challenge. Other challenges include the conditions that lead to health market failure, and
dysfunctions in the referral system.

WAY FORWARD

The way forward includes improving health market regulation through developing the family practice
and referral system, improving sustainable financing and financial support of patients, developing
quality and coverage of health services, developing social partnerships, people-centered healthcare
and inter-sectoral collaboration, and developing plans to control health risk factors and address the
social determinants of health.

REFERENCES

1. King M. *An Iranian Experiment in Primary Health Care: The West Azerbaijan Project.* New York: Oxford University Press; 1983.
2. Shadpour K. *The PHC Experience in Iran.* Tehran: UNICEF; 1994.
3. Pileroudi C. *The District Primary Health Care Networks in Iran.* 2nd ed. Tehran: UNICEF; 1999.
4. Rahbar MR, Ahmadi M. Lessons learnt from the model of instructional system for training community health
   workers in Rural HHs of Iran. *Iran Red Crescent Medical Journal.* 2015;17(2): e2145.
5. Ministry of Health and Medical Education (MoHME). *Health Network Standards.* 2017.
6. MoHME. *Evaluation Study of Family Physician Programme in Rural Areas and Cities under 20 Thousand Population.* Tehran: Noavaran Sina Press; 2013.
7. MoHME. *Executive Order for Family Practice and Rural Health Insurance.* 2017.
8. Ministry of Health and Medical Education of Iran. *Educational programme of Master of Family Medicine for
   General Practitioners.* Approved 2008.

CHAPTER 18

Iraq

Abdul Munem Al Dabbagh, Ghaith Sabri Mohammed, and Thamer Al Hilfi

Total number of PHC facilities	2600
Number of general practitioners working in public PHC facilities	2362*
Number of certified family physicians working in PHC facilities	350
Average number of family physician graduates/year	80–90
Number of medical schools	27
Number of family medicine departments	27

* Excluding the Kurdistan Region.

INTRODUCTION

Most donor attention concerned with rebuilding health services in Iraq, following the invasion in 2003, has focused on the problems of hospitals. Interest in primary health-care services has come about mainly in the past 10 years.[1] Essential health service packages (EHSP) are well integrated at the level of the main healthcare centres which are managed mostly by well-trained general practitioners (GPs) and in some cases by certified family physicians; however, these services are not well integrated at the level of health sub-centres, which are managed by medical auxiliaries whose sole duty is to manage acute emergencies.

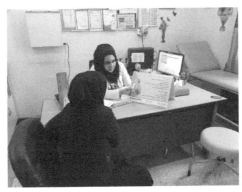

Antenatal care

230 healthcare centres follow the family medicine model with well-established family files, referral systems, and ongoing training programmes.[2] Nine centres have been chosen by the World Health Organization to follow the family health practice approach and are using an electronic health information system; they are under strict quality assurance and accreditation. There is widespread satisfaction with primary health-care services, and levels do not differ appreciably between the public and private sectors. The public sector PHCC services are preferentially used by poorer populations to whom they are important providers. PHCC services are free, with little evidence of informal payments to providers.[3]

Family practice is linked with other initiatives like hospitals and secondary care specialists through many channels such as: [1] A referral system by which family physicians establish contact with hospital doctors (secondary care doctors), receive feedback from them, and adapt the management of their patients collaboratively, [2] Fellowship training for family medicine students offered in some of the training hospitals, [3] Frequent joint scientific activities conducted within the training programmes of the family health centres, inviting secondary care physicians to discuss recent advances and updates in their specialties.

KEY CHALLENGES

The key challenges facing family health practice can be summarized in the following:[4,5]

1. Health personnel are paid equally by the government irrespective of variable workload, which creates a feeling of lack of fairness among health workers.
2. There is a huge gap between available government funding and what is required.
3. There is poor community awareness about family medicine.
4. There is poor motivation for junior doctors and GPs to pursue family medicine as a specialty.

WAY FORWARD

Two successful examples of health facilities implementing family practice are:

- The improvement in the vaccination coverage rate to reach up to 98% of targets, for example, Bab Al Moathem Family Health Centre.
- The increase in the number of people screened for hypertension and diabetes, to involve almost all those targeted.

The Ministry of Health is supporting the expansion of family practice by increasing the number of primary care centres using the family practice approach, and increasing the number of family doctors after academic training. The reasons for the limited production of family physicians in Iraq are: [1] There is only one Iraqi residency programme in family medicine which is capable of graduating no more than 30 to 40 candidates per year. Since starting in 1995, the number of certified family physicians graduated from this programme has not exceeded 200 candidates. [2] The number of Iraqi Arab Board Residency Programme graduates, since 2008, is 150. [3] Emigration and "brain drain" have added to the shortage of available family physicians.

REFERENCES

1. Ministry of Health, Government of Iraq. Health systems based on primary health care in Iraq. *International Conference on Primary Health Care.* 2008. Doha, Qatar.
2. Ministry of Health, Government of Iraq, DG of Public Health. Personal communication.
3. Burnham G, et al. Perceptions and utilization of primary health care services in Iraq: findings from a national household survey. *BMC International Health and Human Rights,* 2011; 11: 15. Available from: https://bmcinthealthhumrights.biomedcentral.com/articles/10.1186/1472-698X-11-15.
4. Ahmed SM. Expectations of physicians working in Erbil city about the role of family medicine practice. *WONCA World Conference.* Prague. 2013.
5. Issa S. Family doctors' satisfaction: a sample from Baghdad. *Iraqi Postgraduate Medical Journal,* 2016; 109 (3): 15–18.

CHAPTER 19

Jordan

Oraib Alsmadi, Mohammed Rasoul Tarawneh,
and May Hani Al Hadidi

	Ministry of Health (MoH)	Royal Medical Services (RMS)	Universities	UNRWA
Total number of PHC facilities	Comprehensive: 102 Primary: 377 Village: 187	12	4	25
Average number of family physician graduates/year	20 since 1993	2–3 since 1985	4–5 since 1999	0
Number of general practitioners working in public PHC facilities	1645			
Number of certified family physicians working in PHC facilities	115 (total of 210 are working in MoH)			
Number of medical schools	6			
Number of family medicine departments	3			

UNRWA: United Nations Relief and Works Agency for Palestine Refugees in the Near East

INTRODUCTION

The government goal is to provide universal health coverage to the entire population. According to the 2015 census, 68% of the population had health insurance, with 8.5% insured by more than one party. MoH insurance is the most prevalent, covering 44.5% of the population. A further 38% of the population is insured through RMS, and 17.5% of Jordanians are insured by university hospitals and the private sector.[1]

All health centres have a well-defined catchment area as a requirement for accreditation. However, because the health system in Jordan is composed of different sectors with no link between them, there is often duplication of medical records, and sometimes the catchment area for a given PHC facility cannot be easily determined.

Guidelines are available at all health facilities; however, they are not updated, and treatment protocols are not accessible to all staff. There are written training plans included in directorate operational

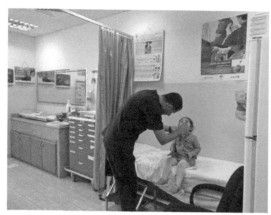

A physician examines a patient

plans; however, some of these plans are not implemented due to financial challenges. The accreditation programme in Jordan has been implemented in MoH PHC settings since 2010. All health centres are using a personal identification number for medical records. The principle of each family being assigned to one specific family doctor or GP is not applied.

The national health strategy 2016–2020 proposes two main ways to achieve universal health coverage: [1] The long-term solution is to increase the production of family physicians.[2,3] [2] The short-term solution is to decrease the gap in producing family physicians by improving the capacities of GPs in the public sector by providing them with online training.

KEY CHALLENGES FOR THE IMPLEMENTATION OF FAMILY PRACTICE[4]

Challenges include: [1] Policy makers with limited awareness of the concept of family practice, [2] Poor logistics management and distribution of health facilities and workforce, [3] Lack of public-private partnerships, [4] Shortage of resources and incentives to ensure proper implementation, [5] Failure of existing training programmes to meet the enormous need for family physicians, [6] Limited legal and financial support to implement family practice.

WAY FORWARD

Initiatives include: [1] Maintain high-level political commitment, [2] Restructure the health system to accommodate trained and certified family physicians, [3] Ensure exposure of medical students to family medicine at the undergraduate level, [4] Ensure availability of on-job capacity building short courses for practising GPs, [5] Support the active engagement of the private sector, [6] Focus on client satisfaction and community perception of family practice, [7] Develop a national roadmap to enhance family practice.

REFERENCES

1. National Health Reform, Jordan. 2018.
2. WHO EMRO, 63rd RC 2016. *Scaling up family practice: progressing towards universal health coverage.* EM/RC63/Tech.Disc.1. Available from: http://www.emro.who.int/about-who/rc63/documentation.html.
3. WHO EMRO, 63rd RC 2016. *Scaling up family practice: progressing towards universal health coverage.* Available from: http://applications.emro.who.int/docs/RC63_Resolutions_2016_R2_19197_EN.pdf?ua=1.
4. WHO EMRO. *Report on the Regional consultation on strengthening service provision through the family practice approach.* Cairo, Egypt, November 2014. WHO-EM/PHC/165/E. Available from: http://apps.who.int/iris/bitstream/handle/10665/253400/IC_meet_rep_2015_EN_16267.pdf?sequence=1&isAllowed=y.

CHAPTER 20

Kuwait

Huda Al-Duwaisan and Fatemah Ahmed Bendhafari

Total number of PHC facilities	103
Number of general practitioners working in public PHC facilities	832
Number of certified family physicians working in PHC facilities	194
Number of certified family physicians in PHC facilities	410
Average number of family physician graduates/year	35

INTRODUCTION

In the six health regions of Kuwait, primary health care centres (PHCCs) provide general, maternal and child, diabetic, and dental clinics. The centres also offer preventive care and school health services. Recently, mental health care services have also been added. In addition, medical records and data are computerized, and it is planned that they will be connected to the secondary and tertiary hospital network. Currently, the total number of PHCCs under the Ministry of Health (MoH) is 103, and these are distributed among all regions. Some of these centres apply the 13 elements of family medicine; others vary in this application, which leads to having both family and general health centres. Each centre provides health services for a population of about 40,000. The services provided are general practice and family medicine, maternal health, child health, dental services, vaccination, and preventive health services. The PHCCs also include diabetic care clinics, chronic disease follow-up, mental health clinics, laboratories, pharmacies, X-ray facilities, and nursing. There are also well-baby clinics and smoking cessation clinics. All health centres include walk-in clinics and recently a system for an appointment-based general clinic was introduced in a family health centre as a pilot.

The drug list available in PHCC pharmacies has been expanded recently to include new medications. The list now includes more than 200 different medications for paediatrics, adults, and geriatrics. The expansion also includes medications for chronic diseases which reduces the burden on central hospitals.

PHC facilities use the electronic file system, Primary Care Information System, for registering patient health information. The system includes risk factors for chronic non-communicable diseases. Currently it covers all PHCCs and linking the system with hospitals will be implemented soon. Primary and family health-care centres follow treatment protocols, work policies, and quality standards according to World Health Organization guidelines. Applying quality protocols to get international accreditation has been started in collaboration with the Canadian Accreditation Council. A 5-year family medicine residency program was established in 1983 in affiliation with the Royal College of General Practitioners in the United Kingdom.

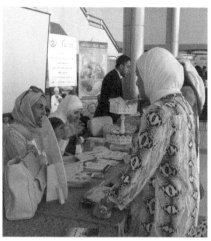

Open day for community, Yarmouk Centre

KEY CHALLENGES

Currently, most primary care services in Kuwait are provided by general practitioners (GPs), representing 64% of the total number of doctors working in primary care. Qualified family physicians comprise the remaining 36%. One of the main challenges in health service delivery is to reduce the waiting time for patients, due to high patient load and over-extension of medical staff. To overcome this, the government is planning to build more hospitals and PHCCs, renovate and build more medical laboratories, and expand dental clinics, as part of the 2015–2019 national development plan.[1] Other challenges include: [1] The need for systematic assessment of the quality of services delivered. [2] Improving referral and follow-up systems. [3] Implementing continuous training and development of health promotion staff. [4] Strengthening home-based and community-based care and community health promotion.

WAY FORWARD

The State of Kuwait continues its endeavours to follow best practice in sustaining primary health care and family medicine practice. The effective introduction of new initiatives relies on champions in PHCCs and within the MoH. As proven in the last two decades, collaborating with international partners is a major pillar contributing to a high level of success. Kuwait will continue efforts to adopt strategies and policies of the World Health Organization and the World Organization of Family Doctors (WONCA). The Supreme Council of Planning has developed a framework for the five-year national plan for all ministries, including the Ministry of Health.[2] The strategic priority areas in national health services that are relevant to primary health care are: [1] Establishing a family practice-based PHC approach across the country. [2] Ensuring interoperable electronic health records across care interfaces. [3] Developing health service research capacity to enable continuous cycles of evaluation and improvement.

REFERENCES

1. *Kuwait National Development Plan 2035.* Available from: http://www.newkuwait.gov.kw/en/plan/ [September 22, 2018].
2. World Health Organization Report 2017. *Development of a New National Health Sector Strategy for the State of Kuwait (2018–2022).*

The authors acknowledge the support of Ms. Hayfaa Almudhaf in data collection and layout design of this chapter.

CHAPTER 21

Lebanon

Walid Ammar and Alissar Rady

Total number of PHC facilities	205 PHC centres in the National MoPH network, out of total 1100 dispensaries*
Number of general practitioners working in public PHC facilities**	Not Available
Number of certified family physicians working in PHC facilities	31 (in 2017)
Average number of family physicians graduates/year	10
Number of medical schools	6
Number of family medicine departments	2

* More than 95% of PHC centres are owned and managed by non-governmental organizations (NGOs); very few are owned or managed by the Ministry of Public Health (MoPH) or the Ministry of Social Affairs (MoSA).
** The number of GPs fluctuates as there is high turnover.

INTRODUCTION

Over the past two decades, the health system in Lebanon has been characterized by a longstanding public–private partnership, a dynamic civil society, a flourishing private sector, and a public sector that is progressively regaining its leadership and regulatory role. The Ministry of Public Health (MoPH) covers hospital stays and expensive medicines for people who are not insured through the program on catastrophic illnesses. The National Social Security Fund and the Government Employee Funds cover around 40% of the population; private insurance covers around 8%. For the 52% of the population that is not covered by health insurance, health services are purchased by the MoPH from the private and public sectors. The MoPH purchases health services from private hospitals, based on a quota and flat rates, through contractual agreements. The MoPH partially subsidizes public hospitals, and also purchases services from them. The MoPH, through in-kind contribution of medicines, vaccines, and trainings, also supports PHC services[1].

Over the past three decades, the MoPH has developed options for provider payment reforms in ambulatory care, and has initiated a system of accreditation for PHC including standard setting guidelines, as well as requirements for physical facilities, workforce, equipment, and operational systems. It also has established a national network of PHC centres that has progressively expanded over the years to cover most geographical areas in the country, with more focus on areas with vulnerable populations. The national network of PHCs provides essential drugs and essential health services, such as paediatrics, family medicine, oral health, reproductive health, cardiology, and vaccination.

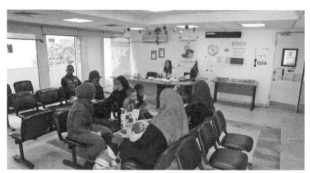
Patients in PHC centre

The MoPH has initiated work on an accreditation mechanism for primary health care corporations, to monitor and ensure quality[2].

KEY CHALLENGES

[1] Promoting family medicine: Attracting general practitioners (GPs) to get formal training in family medicine is a main barrier to introducing the family medicine/people-centred approach. Lebanon has no regulations limiting the number of specialists, or determining the distribution of doctors within specialties and geographic areas. [2] Adapting health service delivery to a family practice approach in PHCs: The current service delivery model through the PHC network of the MoPH is not fully adapted to the role of the family doctor as described in the people-centred approach. The family doctor has limited decision-making authority in the organization of health care.[3] [3] Changing the culture of specialty care: access to specialty care is readily available, and promoting basic family practice comprehensive care requires effort. It needs pre-paid services and regulations for third party payers. [4] Getting stakeholder buy in for the integration of family physicians: With the adoption of the family medicine approach, specialists stand to experience reduction in caseloads in private clinics and loss of income. Neutralizing their opposition to the family medicine approach is an important challenge.

WAY FORWARD

Despite the challenges and limitations, there is a strong momentum for moving forward to reinforce PHC. It requires a paradigm shift for family physicians to be at the heart of a people-centred PHC system. There is ample room for more stakeholders to actively participate in this shift. The following are the main recommendations: [1] To open the door to private practice centres/family physicians' clinics to contribute to the primary care effort and to encourage the MoPH to experiment with capitation schemes. [2] To work towards PHC through a more comprehensive approach, such as the development of the healthy cities/healthy villages concepts. [3] To reposition the family physician at the centre of a gatekeeping mechanism within PHC. [4] To supervise a clear referral system, and to oversee community-oriented interventions.

REFERENCES

1. Ministry of Public Health. Strategic Plan for the medium term (2016 to 2020). Lebanon; 2016. Available from: https://www.moph.gov.lb/userfiles/files/%D9%90Announcement/Final-StrategicPlanHealth2017. pdf [Accessed 19 April 2018].
2. Ministry of Public Health. Accreditation of primary health care centers and quality of care; 2016.
3. Helou, M, Rizk, GA. State of family medicine practice in Lebanon. *Journal of Family Medicine and Primary Care*, 2016;5(1):51–5. Available from: https://www.ncbi.nlm.nih.gov/pubmed/27453843 [Accessed 22 September 2018].

CHAPTER 22

Libya

Syed Jaffar Hussain

Total number of PHC facilities	1355, of which 273 are closed as a result of the conflict
Number of general practitioners working in public PHC facilities	2135
Number of certified family physicians working in PHC facilities	30
Average number of family physician graduates/year	10
Number of medical schools	14
Number of family medicine departments	10

INTRODUCTION

Armed conflict has disrupted the provision of most of the essential health services needed by Libyans, especially the vulnerable. Without enough supplies, manpower, or electricity, many medical centres and private hospitals in conflict-affected areas have been closed, making it difficult for citizens to receive the health care they need. The recent assessment shows that 17 hospitals and 273 primary health-care facilities are closed.[1] Primary health care services are delivered through a wide network of 1355 PHC facilities (including health care units, health care centres, polyclinics). Of these, 20% were closed in 2017[1]. PHC services are perceived by many Libyans to have little to offer patients and, as a result, people tend to bypass the PHC level because of the limited quality of services; they find their way directly to the out-patient clinics or emergency services of secondary or tertiary care hospitals. Many PHC centres have no full-time doctors, and when they do, the doctors are usually young and not very experienced.

The level of functioning health centres and units varies greatly between Shabiat and Tripoli, which has the greatest number of functioning facilities. One in-depth analysis shows that 70% of the medicines from the essential medicine list were not available: doctors encouraged patients to buy medicine privately or to shop around in other centres, polyclinics, or hospitals. Staff capacity is weak: none had trained in family medicine, they had no supervision, and were not involved in any continuing professional development. There are no electronic or paper medical records in most facilities that keep essential information on people in their catchment areas. PHC facilities lack standardized design and have no essential list of the equipment and laboratory facilities that enable the facility to deliver high-quality care. It is believed by many that, for any serious health problem, the outcome of using the PHC would be referral, so skipping PHC speeds up the process.

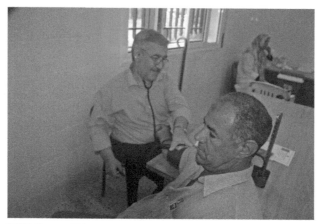

PHC Centre, Tajoura

KEY CHALLENGES

Attempts to modernize health service delivery are facing serious security, political, financial, workforce, and "resistance-to-change" obstacles. Currently, health services are severely challenged. The health system is weak and its overall performance has limitations, including:[2] [1] Lack of a technical health policy and planning functions inside the planning department. [2] Overall weak institutional capacity to plan and implement health programmes at national and sub-national levels. [3] Inadequate and fragmented national health information systems in areas of data required for decision making, ICT infrastructure, and the development of e-records for the health sector. [4] The absence of a health-care financing policy and options for universal coverage schemes. [5] An unclear national human resources development plan, policy, and strategy, and lack of a comprehensive system for continuous professional development.

The key challenges to family practice include: [1] The small number of family physicians graduating each year. [2] No dedicated fund for the implementation of family practice service delivery. [3] No approved professional career for family physicians. [4] Family physicians are considered a threat to other specialties. [5] Lack of coordination between the Ministry of Health (MoH) and the Ministry of Health Education. [6] Little demand from the community for family physicians. [7] During the current crisis, family practice is not one of the top priorities of MoH.

WAY FORWARD

Libya has adopted the approach of improving primary health care through incremental strengthening of the family health model. There is political commitment to scale-up family medicine despite the enormous challenges and the disruption of the health system, with some financial allocations for the national programme. The family health model is adopting an overall reform agenda so that: [1] The MoH is responsible for all primary care service and provision is free to all those working and living in Libya. [2] The government does not license any primary care provider who is not part of MoH services (through direct or contractual service) to ensure equity and maintain the quality, integrity, and comprehensiveness of the service. [3] The MoH is exploring incentives needed to attract high-calibre health professionals to PHC, including family medicine training.

REFERENCES

1. World Health Organization. The Service Availability and Readiness Assessment survey in Libya. 2017 (SARA). Available from: http://www.who.int/hac/crises/lby/en/ [Accessed 20 April 2018].
2. 2017 Review of Health Sector in Libya. https://reliefweb. int/report/Libya /2017-review-health-sector-libya

CHAPTER 23

Morocco

Amina Sahel and Hafid Hachri

Total number of PHC facilities	2759 (760 managed by nurses in rural areas)[1]
Number of general practitioners working in public PHC facilities	3100
Number of certified family physicians working in PHC facilities	45
Average number of family physician graduates/year	40
Number of medical schools	5 public, 2 private

INTRODUCTION

As a signatory of the Alma-Ata Declaration, Morocco has included its Primary Health Care (PHC) strategy in its priorities for governmental action for health. Morocco's first five-year plan for PHC spanned the period 1981 to 1985. Several sectoral projects targeting PHC development were launched with the support of technical and financial partners. These projects made significant contributions to the improvement of health coverage, to the standardization of the approach to coverage and to the restructuring of health programmes.

The coverage made available to the population by primary health-care facilities (PHCFs) has improved significantly. The number of PHCFs rose from 1653 in 1990 to 2689 in 2014,[1] and to 2759 in 2015, a growth of 72% in 25 years.[2] Overall service was improved by 19%, with the ratio of facilities to inhabitants increasing from 1:14,600 in 1990, to 1:11,600 in 2015 (with figures ranging from a maximum of 1:4,400 to a minimum of 1:19,750). The ratio of nurses to the population changed little between 2007 and 2011 (from 1:3267 in 2009 to 1:3327 in 2011), while the coverage provided by general practitioners (GPs) in the public sector in the PHCFs fell from 1.01:10,000 to 0.94:10,000 inhabitants, with even less coverage in rural areas.

Despite the efforts made by the Ministry of Health (MoH) in terms of building PHCFs, the percentage of the population living more than six kilometers from any such facility has remained high at 43%, and mobile coverage remains a valuable alternative.

The health services package provided is defined at the national level and by type of PHCF. In view of the ongoing epidemiological and demographic transition in Morocco, this health services package has been remodeled. [3] The current health services package includes coverage for chronic diseases, notably cardiovascular diseases and diabetes, as well as screening for breast and cervical cancer. Recently, the health services package has been reviewed and redefined as part of a project to reinforce the health-care system. With the exception of emergencies, the transfer from one level to another is through the referral system. The information system is fragmented, oriented towards

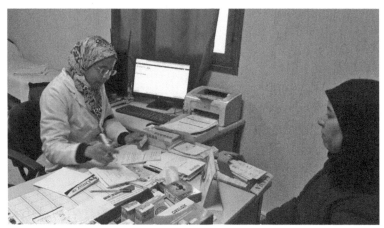

Physician with a patient in a PHC facility

vertical health programmes, and not focused on patients and their families. The MoH has introduced a range of quality measures to instill a culture of quality in the PHCFs.

KEY CHALLENGES FOR IMPLEMENTATION OF FAMILY PRACTICE

Challenges include: [1] Weak political commitment, given that, to date, medical studies have not been reformed to introduce the specialty of family medicine into the country's faculties of medicine. Moreover, the MoH has not officially announced its reform of PHC based on family practice. [2] Lack of training of family doctors. [3] Insufficient regulation and financial support to implement family practice. [4] Absence of registration of the population with PHC doctors. [5] Inadequate system of orientation and a lack of feedback mechanisms. [6] Insufficient private sector commitment and involvement. [7] Community dissatisfaction with public PHC services.

WAY FORWARD

The political commitment of the MoH in favour of the promotion of family practice has been embodied in the national health strategy for 2012 to 2016 and in the new sectoral action plan for 2019 to 2025 which calls for the development of PHC and a revised role for GPs in the implementation of the nation's family and community health training programme. This political commitment should be strengthened by the commitment of other stakeholders involved in the development of family practice, such as faculties of medicine, the Medical Syndicate, and the Ministry of Finance. The MoH has issued a draft decree for partnerships with private GPs, specialists, pharmacists, and dental surgeons which allows contractual agreements to work on a part-time basis in public health facilities, according to availability and the required skills in each health territory. This public–private partnership has been expanded by the involvement of the private sector in strategies and programmes to address a range of priority health issues.

REFERENCES

1. Ministry of Health, Morocco. *Sectoral Strategy for Health 2012–2016*. Available from: https://www.mindbank.info/item/3714 [Accessed 22 September 2018].
2. Ministry of Health, Morocco. *Hospitals and Ambulatory Health Department Database*. 2017.
3. Ministry of Health, Morocco. *Health Coverage by the Basic Health Care Network. Methodological Guide for the Production of an Extension Plan*. 1990.

CHAPTER 24

Oman

Said Al Lamki and Ahmed Salim Saif Al-Mandhari

Total number of PHC facilities	235
Number of general practitioners working in public PHC facilities	3837
Number of certified family physicians working in PHC facilities	143
Average number of family physician graduates/year	16–20
Number of medical schools	2
Number of family medicine departments	2

INTRODUCTION

The primary care service delivery system is well-established and is based on clear principles. The size and type of structures of PHC facilities depend on the population, distance from other referral centres/hospitals, and logistics.[1]

PHC facilities are generally classified as health centres, extended health centres (with delivery facility), polyclinics, and local hospitals.

PHC facilities are staffed with general practitioners, nurses, pharmacists, assistant pharmacists, dentists, dental assistant nurses, lab technicians, radiographers, health educators, dieticians, medical orderlies, medical record clerks, and drivers.

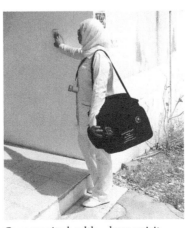

Community health – home visit

The current density of family physicians in Oman is 0.3/10,000 population, which is lower than the rate recommended by the Ministry of Health (MoH) (2/10,000 population, based on recommendations of the Gulf Cooperation Council Ministers Qarar, Kuwait 2007).[2] The density of nurses is below the European standard of 65/100,000 population.[3]

The health centres are considered the first contact point for all citizens and residents. These centres are supported by Wilayat (governorate), local, and regional referral hospitals.

From the primary health-care centre/facility, patients are referred to a higher level of care with more advanced services such as in-patient services, surgery, or intensive care.

In general, patients are referred from a health centre to the local hospital or polyclinic. A comprehensive manual was developed to govern and guide the process of referral and back referral (2004). Some of these manuals have not been updated since then.

KEY CHALLENGES

Despite the above-mentioned achievements, there are several challenges facing PHC: [1] Most PHC facilities have too little space, with inadequate consultation rooms and little emergency space and equipment. [2] Inadequate support services including laboratory, imaging services, diagnostic services, and equipment. [3] Shortage of skilled health-care workers such as family physicians. [4] Increasing magnitude of chronic diseases. [5] Newly emerging global public health threats.

WAY FORWARD

In the past, communicable diseases caused substantial morbidity and mortality in Oman, but in recent years lifestyle-related or non-communicable diseases (NCDs) and the changing age structure of the population have begun to reveal new morbidity patterns. The results of the National Health Survey 2000, conducted by the MoH, portrayed a worrisome picture of the risk factors for NCDs. The morbidity statistics in 2011 for MoH health facilities show that about 49.9% of all out-patient visits, and 37.6% of hospital admissions, are for NCDs[3]. This has led to an important transformation in the PHC programs, with a shift in focus towards NCDs and PHC services such as: [1] Mini-diabetes clinics: A mini-diabetes clinic is available in almost every health centre. This service provides the basic medications for diabetes management.[4] [2] Services for diabetic foot care: Since 2008, there has been structured health education on diabetic foot care, with a guideline for diabetic foot assessment and management.[5] [3] Services for hypertensive patients: Doctors and nurses in PHC settings have been trained to diagnose and treat patients with hypertension. [4] Services for mental illness: Integrating mental health services into primary care is the most viable way of ensuring that people have access to the mental health care they need. [5] NCD screening programme: This programme is directed towards screening of those above 40 years for early detection and prevention of NCD, mainly hypertension, diabetes, hyperlipidaemia, obesity, and renal disease. [6] Elderly care: This provides comprehensive assessment of elder patients and suitable interventions like clinical intervention, physiotherapy provided by mobile physiotherapy units, social interventions and referral services.

REFERENCES

1. Primary health care vision 2050 documents presented in health care vision of Oman 2050 conference. May 2012.
2. MoH, Sultanate of Oman. 8th Five-Year Plan for Health Development, 2011–2015. Available from: http://www.nationalplanningcycles.org/sites/default/files/country_docs/Oman/five_year_plan_for_health_development_2011-2015.pdf [Accessed 17 April 2018].
3. MoH, Sultanate of Oman, 2016. Annual Health Report 2016.
4. International Diabetes Federation IDF Diabetes Atlas (Eighth edition). 2017. Available from: http://www.diabetesatlas.org/ [Accessed 17 April 2018].
5. Al-Lawati, JA, Al-Riyami, AM, Mohammed, AJ, Jousilahti, P. Increasing prevalence of diabetes mellitus in Oman. *Diabetic Medicine.* 2002, 19 (11): 954–957. Available from: https://onlinelibrary.wiley.com/doi/pdf/10.1046/j.1464-5491.2002.00818.x [17 April 2018].

CHAPTER 25

Pakistan

Waris Qidwai, Marie Andrades, Zia UlHaq, and Kashmira Nanji

Total number of PHC facilities	11,530
Number of general practitioners (GPs) working in public PHC facilities	Data is not available
Number of certified family physicians (FPs) working in PHC facilities	18
Average number of family physician graduates/year	Data is not available
Number of medical schools*	107
Number of family medicine departments	7

*41 public and 66 private

INTRODUCTION

Primary health-care services are both community and facility-based. Community health workers include lady health workers (LHWs), community midwives, vaccinators, and sanitary inspectors.[1] Approximately 92,900 LHWs (0.43 per 1000 population) provide PHC services at the community level. Facility-based services are offered via a network of civil dispensaries, basic health units, and rural health centres.[2] The temporal aspects of service delivery may differ from facility to facility.

As a path to achieve universal health care, the federal and provincial governments have launched social health protection initiatives to provide financial protection for their populations. It is estimated that the private sector provides 70–80% of out-patient services.[3] Provision of family planning services is attempted at the PHC facility and community level including counselling on birth spacing, adopting modern techniques, and empowering women to adopt family planning. Routine immunization, public health emergency and disaster preparedness, disability, mental health, and oral health are the essential components of PHC services. Limited studies have been conducted to assess the satisfaction of quality of service delivery from PHC. The available literature shows that patients are more satisfied with private hospitals than the public sector. The rates of dissatisfaction with the public sector are as high as 80%.

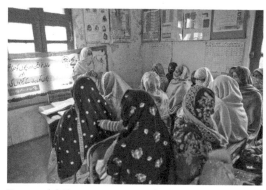

Postnatal follow-up at a PHC facility

KEY CHALLENGES

The total number of PHC facilities is 11,530, which are managed by GPs. However, only 18 facilities are run by a certified FP. Out of 107 medical schools there are only four Family Medicine departments. Availability of the Essential Health Service Package varies from province to province depending on its location. Currently, there is no well-organized Family Practice system. Prevention is not the primary focus, leading to lack of integration into the health system. NCDs, geriatric care, and mental health issues have not been made a part of the health services package. The health information and surveillance system needs strengthening as most information received is inaccurate and unused. Other challenges include the perceived threat by specialists who consider the frontline family health-care model to be a threat to their practice. Public-private partnerships have been attempted as a new model of health service in family practice, but these have not been very successful as there is a lack of clarity concerning the mechanism for contracting with the private sector and a lack of clearly outlined indicators of performance and outcomes. There are over 168,000 registered medical doctors; presuming even half are practicing as GPs, this is a huge number and they need to be trained to enhance their competencies as FPs.

WAY FORWARD

Family practice can play a critical role in improving health indicators for any country. The government has not previously shown the will to make it an integral part of the health system. The National Health Vision 2016–2020 has articulated eight thematic pillars for the health system. These include health financing, health service delivery, human resources, health information systems, governance, essential medicines and technology, cross-sectoral linkages, and global health responsibilities.

In order for family practice to succeed in terms of affordability, access, and quality of care, there must be reaching out to the community through home health-care services and a strong link with secondary and tertiary care centres. There is a need to link family practice centres with the other non-governmental organizations (NGOs) already working in the field, in order to fill in the gaps in services where required. Linkages with private quality maternity homes would help in providing obstetric care. In addition, government health insurance schemes need to be linked with family practice to make services affordable for the population.

REFERENCES

1. Sixth Five-Year Plan 1978–1983, Chapter 19: Towards a Comprehensive National Coverage. Planning Commission, Government of Pakistan. Available from: http://www.pakistan.gov.pk/ministries/planninganddevelopment-ministry/index.htm [Dec, 2017].
2. Hafeez A, Mohamud BK, Shiekh MR, Shah SAI, Jooma R. Lady health workers programme in Pakistan: challenges, achievements and the way forward. *JPMA*, 2011; 61(3): 210.
3. Malik MA, Gul W, Iqbal SP, Abrejo F. Cost of primary health care in Pakistan. *Journal of Ayub Medical College Abbottabad*, 2015; 27(1): 88–92.

CHAPTER 26

Palestine

Rand Salman, Gerald Rockenschaub, and Asa'd Ramlawi

Indicator	Region		Total
	West Bank	**Gaza Strip**	
PHC facilities (MoH, UNRWA, NGOs, and military services)	587	152	739
General practitioners	4671	1745	6416
General practitioners working in PHC public facilities of MoH	400	153	553
Certified family physicians working in PHC facilities	25 within MoH PHC	21 in MoH PHC,15 in UNRWA	61
Family physician graduates/year (average)	3–5 per year	Not reported	
Medical schools	2 (An-Najah and Al-Quds University)	2 (Islamic University and a branch of Al-Quds University)	4
Family medicine departments	1 (An-Najah University)	1 (Al-Azhar University)	2
MoH family medicine training centres	3	3	6

INTRODUCTION

Primary health-care services in Palestine are provided by the Ministry of Health (MoH), non-governmental organizations (NGOs), the United Nations Relief and Works Agency (UNRWA), military medical services, and the private sector.[1] There are 4671 general practitioners working in the West Bank and 1745 GPs working in the Gaza Strip; 400 GPs work in PHC clinics of the MoH in the West Bank and 153 in MoH clinics in Gaza. The PHC system in Palestine suffers from overall staffing constraints with a shortage of trained and specialized family physicians. The essential health services package included in the basic services package covers services for reproductive health, newborn and child health, an expanded programme of immunization, communicable diseases, NCD, general clinic services, mental health, behavioural change communication, first aid, dental health, nutrition, laboratory services, and pharmaceutical services. Some or all of these services are available at PHC centres. The PHC services provided by the MoH do not always cover all of the services included in an adequately defined Essential Health Service Package. Shortages of essential medicines, and limited accessibility resulting from restricted working hours, remain of concern. The essential drugs list, which was developed in the year 2000, includes some 500 essential pharmaceuticals, including 210 items for PHC services. There is limited monitoring to ensure the prescribed medications are aligned with the established treatment protocols. Family practice services are provided by family doctors, supported by a multidisciplinary team. The family practice approach is characterized by comprehensive, continuous, integrated, family, and community-oriented services.

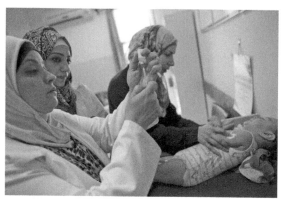

Vaccination in a PHC facility

KEY CHALLENGES

Although adaptations have been introduced to improve the PHC system, there are persistent challenges to continuously enhance service quality through family practice. Gaps remain in dedicated family practice services for rural outreach or to support the health needs of marginalized groups in rural or vulnerable areas. Community participation needs further strengthening. To implement the family practice model, adjustments in three main areas are under consideration:[2] [1] To improve the image and quality of PHC services and strengthen patient–provider relationships [2] To provide more client-friendly organization of services [3] To expand the model and quality of services. These factors are linked to the following specific challenges in the implementation of family practice: limited opening hours of many PHC facilities, lack of a comprehensive patient records system, inadequate emphasis on the gatekeeping role, and the ongoing occupation of the West Bank and the closure of Gaza which leads to chronic shortages of drugs and equipment.

WAY FORWARD

The Palestinian Ministry of Health is fully committed to re-orienting the existing PHC system towards Family Practice (FP). This political step has translated into the establishment of the first Family Medicine postgraduate course in 2010 in the West Bank and in 1990 in Gaza.

The Ministry of Health, is committed to implementing the family practice model including the following seven pillars:[2] [1] Responsible FP teams [2] Registration of patients with a specific FP team [3] Single electronic patient record using a national identification number [4] Introduction of a tailored appointment system to reduce waiting time and increase contact time [5] Repeat prescriptions, rational drug use, and optimizing NCD/chronic disease management [6] Gatekeeping [7] Integrated care.

REFERENCES

1. Palestinian Ministry of Health. Annual report of the Ministry of Health 2016. 2017. Gaza Strip. p. 68.
2. World Health Organization Towards Family Practice (FP) in Palestine (WHO recommendations for developing a Family Practice Strategy). 2017. Palestine. p. 41.

CHAPTER 27

Qatar

Mariam Ali Abdulmalik, Zelaikha Mohsin Al-Wahedi, and Muna Taher Aseel

Total number of PHCC facilities	26
Number of general practitioners working in public PHCC facilities	220
Number of certified family physicians working in PHCC facilities	321
Average number of family physician graduates/year	8
Number of medical schools	2
Number of family medicine departments	1

INTRODUCTION

In Qatar, both public and private facilities provide nationals and residents with primary healthcare services. The Primary Health Care Corporation (PHCC) is the main and largest public-sector provider of primary care services. There are 1.65 million patients registered for PHCC services, of which 1.24 million have been confirmed as active patients. This population base is constantly changing, mainly as short-term expatriate residents enter and leave the country.[1]

Primary health care services are focused on health promotion, prevention, early screening, and disease and continuous care management, and will become more centred on groups of patients defined as "Priority Populations" with the greatest need focused on children and adolescents, women, the ageing population and healthy elderlies, employees, mental health patients, and people with chronic disease.

The PHCC is introducing a family medicine model of care, which is changing the way in which PHCC delivers consultant-led care. The Qatar National Formulary provides a comprehensive reference tool, to manage the increasing range of medicines available, as part of the overall economic and social expansion of the country. The PHCC has a highly skilled and motivated primary care workforce, working in teams and centred on patient and family care. All 23 PHC centres are run by family physicians supported by multidisciplinary teams. A clinical guidelines adoption programme was initiated to ensure appropriate governance of the development of clinical guidelines. The benefits of Clinical Information Systems have been revolutionary for primary care by improving the safety and quality of data capture and retention and enabling easy access to patient information. The PHCC completed its second accreditation survey facilitated by Accreditation Canada International. The Research Section has established an accredited staff research, training, and capacity building programme to boost research capability among family physicians and other frontline staff.

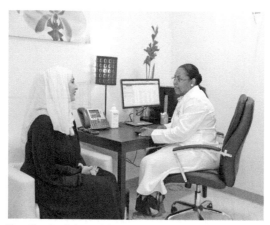

Family physician with patient in PHCC facility

KEY CHALLENGES

A formal evaluation of the family practice pilot is currently underway. Throughout the implementation of the family practice pilot in 2017, several challenges arose, the most significant of these[3] was the cultural acceptance to see the assigned family physician and build continuity of care and continuing care/integrated services support from the wider health system. Although Qatar has made significant advancement in recent years, there are still many challenges faced by the health system. A number of challenges were addressed in national health strategies as well as the PHCC's own Corporate Strategic Plan 2018–2022:[1,2][1] Population changes and complex demographics, [2] Influencing change in a culture based on treating illness, [3] Establishing leadership in prevention and self-care, [4] Local and global staffing constraints, [5] Pace and scale of transformation in the health system, [6] Resistance to change and ever-increasing patient expectations, [7] Need for strengthened integration across the health system.

WAY FORWARD

There is a clear determination to shift the balance from secondary to primary care, and this national commitment is demonstrated in the establishment of PHCC, and supported by the goals outlined in the National Health Strategy (NHS) 2011–16. The NHS provides an overarching strategic vision and direction for health-care delivery, with a clear shift from treatment of illness to prevention and health promotion. This is further strengthened in the NHS 2018–22[1] with clear initiatives dedicated to the delivery of a family medicine model in primary care.

The implementation of a family medicine model across all PHCC facilities is a clear directive of the Mid-Term Review of the National Primary Health Care Strategy 2013–18, and PHCC has committed to mobilizing new health centres with the family practice model and transitioning all existing health centres starting in 2018. The successful piloting, evaluation, and implementation of a family practice model will set the precedent for standardizing primary care services across the health sector. Implementation of a standardized family practice approach to primary care services should be mandated across all public and private sector facilities with performance and quality monitored at a ministerial level.

REFERENCES

1. Ministry of Public Health, Qatar. *National Health Strategy 2018–2022*. 2018. Available from: https://www.moph.gov.qa/HSF/Pages/NHS-18-22.aspx [Accessed 29 March 2018].
2. HI Management Department - PHCC Qatar. December Report, HIM Statistical Monthly Report. *2017*.
3. Primary Health Care Corporation, Family Medicine Project Team, 2017.

CHAPTER 28

Saudi Arabia

Noha Dashash, Lubna A. Al-Ansary, and Ibrahim El-Ziq

Total number of PHC facilities[1]	2400
Number of general practitioners (GPs) working in public PHC facilities[2]	6107
Number of certified family physicians (FPs)[3] working in PHC facilities[2]	636
Average number of family physician (Board and Diploma) graduates/year[2]	100–120
Total family medicine residents enrolled in 2015[2]	226
Number of governmental medical schools	25
Number of private medical schools[4]	6
Number of family medicine departments in medical colleges[2]	25
Number of family medicine programmes within medical colleges or joint postgraduate programmes[2]	18

INTRODUCTION

The Primary Health Care Centres (PHCCs) network covers most of the population and provides comprehensive care for acute and chronic health problems as well as health promotion services, such as health education and immunization for all citizens.[3] There are 2400 PHCCs, 60% of which are in rural areas all over the country. Service is covered by 6107 general practitioners (GPs) and 636 family physicians (FPs). Most FPs are based in cities which includes less than 10% of all PHCCs, whereas rural PHCCs are run by GPs. Recently, the Ministry of Health (MoH) has launched an extensive renovation project to renew all governmental PHCC buildings, thereby transforming them into modern attractive facilities. Radiological services are present in 35% of PHCCs, 61% have laboratories.[2]

Essential drugs are available in most PHCCs. The number of drugs included has doubled over the past few years to include more than 350 items. Referral between PHCCs and hospitals is generally below the desired standard.[4] In order to improve the quality of care provided in PHCCs, the MoH has set an extensive quality control and accreditation programme for all PHCCs. PHC Clinical Practice Guidelines are based on good research evidence of clinical effectiveness. The private sector has shown interest in providing family practice services in the past few years.

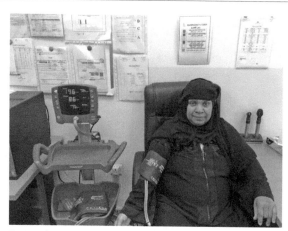

Patient having a periodic checkup

KEY CHALLENGES

Patient satisfaction studies with PHCCs have had conflicting results. A study in Riyadh[5] showed that about 30% of the participants perceive PHCC services as weak or ineffective. With regard to the likelihood of choosing PHCCs as the first choice of health-care service, 75% of the participants admitted that PHCCs are not their first choice. Rural coverage remains a challenge in Saudi Arabia. One of the main challenges in providing optimal primary health-care services, is the lack of certified family physicians. This shortage is not only a local shortage, it is a regional one.

WAY FORWARD

Saudi Arabia is currently undergoing a huge reform. The aim of this transformation is reaching the 2030 vision set by the Crown Prince. Health-care transformation will result in a sustainable health-care system that focuses on the health and wellbeing of people. It comprises seven main themes:[5] model of care, health-care financing, corporatization, private sector participation, governance, e-health, and workforce

The core of health-care transformation is the model of care which incorporates six systems of care: 'Chronic Care', 'Safe Birth', 'Last Phase', 'Planned care', 'Urgent Care' and 'Keep me well'. These focus on activating the people and communities, with the priority being the prevention of disease by several means including screening and health promotion. A great deal of the model of care implementation is carried out by family physicians within PHCCs.

The model of care adopts an integrated, patient-centered, health-care delivery system. In fact, the Saudi Arabian health-care leadership recognizes that the most efficient way to provide high-quality, efficient health care is through effective PHC run by family physicians. This has encouraged the political leadership to support and commit to plans that aim at increasing the number of qualified family physicians.

REFERENCES

1. General Authority for Statistics. *Population Characteristics Surveys.* 2017. Available from: https://www.stats.gov.sa/.
2. Al-Khaldi YM, Al-Ghamdi EA, Al-Mogbil TI, Al-Khashan HI. Family medicine practice in Saudi Arabia: The current situation and proposed strategic directions plan 2020. *Journal of Family and Community Medicine.* 2017;24(3): 156–163. doi:10.4103/jfcm.JFCM_41_17.
3. Primary Healthcare Center Accreditation Program. https://portal.cbahi.gov.sa/english/accreditation-programs/primary-healthcare-center-accreditation-program
4. Ministry of Education. Moe.gov.sa. 2018 Available from: https://www.moe.gov.sa/ (March 2018).
5. Alsakkak MA, Alwahabi SA, Alsalhi HM, Shugdar MA. Outcome of the first Saudi Central Board for Accreditation of Healthcare Institutions (CBAHI) primary health care accreditation cycle in Saudi Arabia. *Saudi Medical Journal.* 2017;38(11): 1132–1136. Available from: doi:10.15537/smj.2017.11.20760.

CHAPTER 29

Somalia

Mona Ahmed Almudhwahi and Abdihamid Ibrahim

Total number of PHC facilities	457
Number of general practitioners working in public PHC facilities	1065 in hospitals only. No doctors working in PHC facilities
Number of certified family physicians working in PHC facilities	Data is not available
Average number of family physician graduates/year	0
Number of medical schools	6*
Number of family medicine departments	1 (Borama University)

* These are the recognized medical schools only.

INTRODUCTION

Somalia's health service delivery is provided through a two-pronged approach. The first is through the Somali Humanitarian Fund (SHF), formerly known as the Common Humanitarian Fund (CHF), or the Humanitarian Response Plan, aimed to deliver relief operations. The second approach is through a recently developed, piloted, and adopted package called the Essential Package of Health Services (EPHS), which was launched in 2014 by the Federal Government of Somalia and aims to improve equitable access to acceptable, affordable, and quality health services. This developmental health process envisages the scaling up of government leadership, management, and service delivery capacity, while sustaining health partners' support, thus averting the transitional funding gap often encountered during a post-conflict period, when the health system is transitioning to recovery, institutional rebuilding and development.

The health worker requirements, and the essential drugs and technologies necessary for implementing the EPHS programmatic interventions, have also been standardized. Health service delivery is structured around the framework of the EPHS.[1] However, it is not being implemented uniformly across the country and covers only nine of the 18 regions, due to factors such as limited resources and security challenges. In the remaining nine regions, health service delivery is inconsistent and dependent on the presence of humanitarian organizations.

The Somali private health sector is a fast-growing sector that is dominating health service provision. Evidence shows that the majority of patients seek help from the private sector, which indicates poor access to public health facilities.

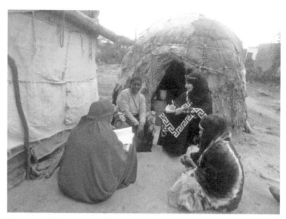

Community outreach

KEY CHALLENGES

The provision of effective service delivery is facing five main challenges. [1] Financing of EPHS: The country's health sector programmes are donor dependent and the government's contribution is less than 2%. [2] Human resources for health: The health workforce is the backbone of the health system and often constitutes the most significant element in the provision of essential and lifesaving health services to the population. [3] Insecurity and access issues: This limits the ability of health sector partners and authorities to scale up health services and ensure equitable health service distribution. [4] Institutional and governance capacities: Prolonged conflict has led to total health system collapse and poor institutional capacity. [5] Regulatory framework for the health sector: Weak regulatory frameworks and limited capacity of law enforcement have contributed to the poor quality of health services.

WAY FORWARD

To improve EPHS implementation five strategic actions are needed.[2,3] [1] Predictable and sustainable financing for the EPHS: The government needs to increase budgetary allocation for EPHS implementation. The current external financing is not only insufficient, but also not sustainable. [2] Enhanced production of a qualified and competent mid-level health workforce: The availability of qualified, competent staff with the right skill mix is at the heart of a revived health sector in Somalia. [3] Strengthened institutional capacity for health authorities at all levels to support government ownership and leadership: International development partners supporting the country's health sector need to invest in building capacity at federal, state, and regional levels to ensure government ownership, leadership, and sustainability of health sector programmes. [4] Scale up and ensuring equitable access to basic health services and moving towards universal health coverage (UHC): For the country to move towards achievement of UHC, and to ensure equity of basic health service delivery, EPHS needs to be scaled up to include nomadic and rural districts of the country. [5] Continuing re-building and improving the regulatory framework to improve quality of health-care services and infrastructure: Since public institutions and universities are weak, a holistic public-private partnership approach, with a well-defined regulatory framework, is required for achievement of UHC in Somalia.

REFERENCES

1. Pearson N, Muschell J. *Essential Package of Health Services Somaliland 2009.* UNICEF. Available from: https://www.unicef.org/somalia/SOM_EssentialSomalilandReport_3_WEB.pdf
2. World Health Organization. *Strategic review of the Somali Health Sector: Challenges and Prioritized Actions. Report of the WHO mission to Somalia.* September 2015.
3. Ministry of Health. *Health Information Management System.* 2012/13/14.

CHAPTER 30

Sudan

Abdalla Sid Ahmed Osman, Eiman Hag, Hind Amin Merghani, and Naeema Al Gasseer

Total number of PHC facilities	6220
Number of general practitioners working in public PHC facilities	Not Available
Number of certified family physicians working in PHC facilities	46
Average number of family physician graduates/year	40 MD, 300 MSc
Number of medical schools	37
Number of family medicine departments	5

INTRODUCTION

Primary health care (PHC) is high on the agenda of ongoing health system reform in Sudan. Currently, PHC coverage is reported to be 95% of the population. However, there is less progress in the coverage by functioning Family Health Centres (FHCs) and Family Health Units (FHUs); by mid-2017 the coverage was 88% and 77% of the population respectively. With increased government commitment and sustainable financing, PHC coverage is expanding to include unreached population groups. According to the Joint Assessment Report 2017, three states reported achieving full functionality of FHUs namely: Gadarif, Sinnar, and River Nile; while two states reported less than 50% functional FHCs namely: Red Sea and South Kordofan; and another two states, namely: North Darfur and Central Darfur have less than 50% of functional FHUs.[1]

Essential health service packages (EHSPs) are fragmented and not unified across providers. The Ministry of Health (MoH) health finance policy sets out a provider/purchaser split.[2]

PHC infrastructure has received great attention from the MoH in recent years. An expansion project started in 2012 and focuses mainly on infrastructure and human resources for health training. The content of the EHSP provided at PHC level is based on the burden of diseases. The finance policy ensures that the National Health Insurance Fund (NHIF) provides the EHSP and the comprehensive package for all the insured population in addition to the poor.[2] The number of health facilities providing the complete EHSP has increased from 24% to 62% between 2011 and 2016.[3] A recent study showed that the availability of essential medicines at public and private health facilities reached 73% and 90% respectively.[4]

Treatment protocols and guidelines are neither unified nor fully implemented. There have been a number of efforts undertaken to strengthen the referral system. Reform in health information is underway to promote more integration and an accreditation council has been established.

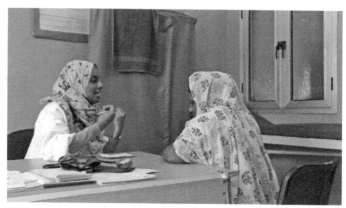
PHC physician with a patient

CHALLENGES

One of the biggest challenges is that the majority of family physician graduates migrate to countries in the Gulf Region and elsewhere, leaving an exceptionally small number of physicians in the country to lead this profession.[4] Although one of the three main objectives targeted by the PHC expansion project is to ensure the quality and sustainability of PHC services, there is no well-functioning quality assurance system in place, and there is a lack of clinical protocols, guidelines, quality standards, and indicators. On the other hand, some strategies and activities have been put in place to improve the quality of PHC services, such as standards for building and rehabilitating the infrastructure and equipment of health facilities, as well as recruitment and training of family physicians and members of family health teams.[3]

WAY FORWARD

The priority of the NHIF in coming years is to enroll all the poor through governmental subsidies. The government increased coverage of the poor from 500,000 to 750,000 to 1 million families during the last three years. Moreover, as an implementation strengthening mechanism, purchasing guidelines have been developed. Additionally, the PHC expansion project is high on the government agenda and is funded by the Ministry of Finance. Political commitment at the national level to family practice has increased during recent years. The higher authority in Sudan is the National Health Coordination Council, chaired by the president of Sudan. This council is committed to universal health coverage (UHC) and has endorsed the family health policy. The MoH is working towards UHC, and implementing the family health approach, through PHC expansion and training of doctors in family medicine in addition to other health staff.[3,5] The family health policy has three main objectives: [1] to strengthen the PHC service delivery system in order to enable the provision of efficient and equitable quality health services; [2] to improve the recognition of the specialty of family medicine, and increase the retention of family physicians; [3] to ensure the production of competent family physicians and allied health workers to provide integrated, people-centred health services at the PHC level.[6]

REFERENCES

1. Federal Ministry of Health. *Joint Assessment Report, Sudan.* 2017.
2. Federal Ministry of Health, Public Health Institute. *Health Finance Policy.* 2015.
3. Federal MoH, Public Health Institute. *Family Medicine in Sudan: A Situation Analysis.* 2015.
4. Federal Ministry of Health, Public Health Institute. The National Health Policy 2017–2030.
5. Federal Ministry of Health, Primary Health Care General Directorate, Expansion Project. *Annual Report 2017.*
6. Federal Ministry of Health. Strengthening Primary Health Care in Sudan through a Family Health Approach: Policy Options. 2016.

CHAPTER 31

Syria

Majid Bitar and Arwa Eissa

The number of primary health-care facilities	1826
Number of general practitioners (GPs) working in public primary health-care facilities	850
The number of specialist family physicians working in primary health-care facilities	100
Average number of family physician graduates/year	8
Number of medical universities or colleges	8
Number of family medicine divisions or departments	2

INTRODUCTION

There is no doubt that the crisis that Syria has undergone for the past seven years, has affected the health sector. Many hospitals and health centres have suffered structural damage in whole or in part. Some of them have gone out of service; others had services reduced or were forced to use neighbouring buildings to provide services. Additionally, public electricity and water supply was disrupted, which often was almost permanent. Many of the Ministry of Health (MoH) vehicles, especially ambulances, were rendered non-operational, because of direct or indirect targeting.

The number of health professionals has shrunk dramatically.[1] Challenges include the difficulty of gaining access to clean water, the damage sewage networks have suffered, overcrowding, especially in shelters, resulting from the arrival of displaced population from unsafe places, food insecurity in varying degrees, and increasing pressure on remaining functioning health centres.

Additionally, the number of those suffering from psychological distress, depression, addiction, and serious mental illness, as well as suicide cases, has doubled. This has seriously worsened the health situation in the country. Vaccination coverage rates have dwindled; multiple cases of malnutrition have been recorded; and polio, measles, and other diseases, especially communicable diseases, have emerged.[2] The essential drug list is regularly updated and reviewed. Treatment protocols are not universally available in health centres. The referral system is currently inactive. The primary health care information system is the routine health information system. The private sector's role in the provision of out-patient services is increasing.

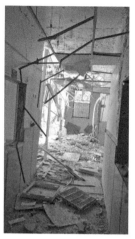

Nowa el Awal Family
Health Centre, Deraa

CHALLENGES

Access to quality services is facing the following significant challenges:[3] [1] Many health centres have been rendered completely out of service, and many others have also been partially affected, with an urgent need to rehabilitate them, [2] Poor capabilities and resources and the consequent impact on the readiness of centres and the quality of services, [3] The number of visitors to some centres has doubled as a result of the population's relocation to safer places, which in turn has made it difficult to provide fair, quality services to all patients, [4] The absence of training of substitutes for those who perform particular services in some health centres. The challenges facing family practice include: [1] The lack of a supportive political decision-making, [2] Lack of MoH support for family medicine specialists, [3] Lack of adequate motivation for skilled family doctors, and the need to work in private clinics as well as in health care facilities, [4] Lack of public or private initiatives to empower or encourage family practice.

WAY FORWARD

The provision of integrated health services in the context of a protracted crisis has a major impact on the health sector, especially on PHC facilities. The priority has been, and remains, to restore basic services, rehabilitate and renovate affected centres, provide human cadres, reassign them, and restore all health coverage rates to what they had been before the crisis. The MoH has continued to provide basic primary health care services even to places that are difficult to reach and out of control. Further, it has carried out and continues to implement vigorous national vaccination campaigns. The MoH provided shelters, across all governorates and regions, with the necessary medical staff, medicines, and the possibility of referral of critical cases. The MoH has developed, since the beginning of the crisis, a strategic plan to provide mental health services and primary psychological care through selected primary health care centres. To assess the current situation and to update the data on the assessment and readiness of health services provided in all health centres, the Service Availability and Readiness Assessment Survey is being conducted in collaboration with the World Health Organization. Work has been underway for more than two years on rehabilitation and restoration of health centres. The MoH has given considerable attention to the issue of infection control through coordination and cooperation with concerned authorities.

REFERENCES

1. Statistical Memorandum of the Directorate of Planning and International Cooperation (2017). Available from: http://www.moh.gov.sy/
2. Epidemiological Bulletins of the WHO for Early Warning Alert and Response System, for the 2017 year. Available from: http://www.emro.who.int/syr/ewars-workshops/ewars-bulletins-2017.html.
3. Regulatory Decision No T/8 (Oct 2017), Integrated Health Centers (Health Centers-Specialized Health Centers), [supplement No 1: Human Resources].

CHAPTER 32

Tunisia

Ali Mtiraoui and Belgacem Sabri

Total number of PHC facilities	2091
Number of general practitioners working in public PHC facilities	5000
Number of certified family physicians working in PHC facilities	150
Average number of family physician graduates/year	80
Number of medical schools	4
Number of family medicine departments	4

INTRODUCTION

The Tunisian health-care system has achieved good health indicators in terms of life expectancy and reduced mortality and morbidity, and compares well with countries of similar income and level of health care expenditure inside and outside the WHO Eastern Mediterranean Region[1].

Health achievements are also caused by improvement of social determinants of health, including education and women's rights, and large social health protection since the independence of the country in late the 1950s.

The bold population policy adopted in the mid-sixties has allowed integration of family planning and reproductive health into primary care settings and helped to control demographic growth.

The health-care system has a strong network of primary care facilities in both the public and private sectors, and focuses on health promotion and prevention. Nearly 50% of physicians are general practitioners (GPs) working in health teams in the public sector and involved in promotive, preventive, curative, rehabilitative and palliative care through national programs managed by the Ministry of Health.

In the private sector GPs work in solo practice, dealing mainly with curative care, and are not fully involved in national health promotion and prevention programs despite efforts made through health education and opportunities for continuing professional development.

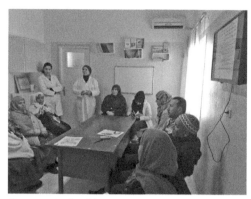

Community health program

CHALLENGES

The Tunisian health system is facing important challenges including advanced epidemiological and demographic transitions, deterioration of many of the social determinants of health, and rising population expectations for access to quality health care while resources are diminishing.

Risk factors are rising, including high prevalence of smoking and substance abuse, obesity, lack of physical activity, inappropriate diet particularly among youth, road traffic accidents and domestic violence. This situation puts additional economic and service delivery pressures on the health system due to the rise of non-communicable and chronic diseases.

Service provision needs to become more community-based focusing on promotion of healthy lifestyles, and on improving the major social determinants of health. Engagement with civil society organizations and coordination with other related sectors remains limited, despite the efforts made after the 2011 revolution[2].

Financial constraints, as a consequence of structural adjustment programs initiated since the late 1980s, have had a negative impact on the availability of health technology and the workforce needed in primary care settings. Opportunities for continuing education and professional development of staff working in first line facilities are also diminishing.

WAY FORWARD

There are opportunities represented by the nation's new constitution protecting the right to health and political commitment to universal health coverage through community-centered primary health care. A law was passed on the development of family medicine reform which began in 2017.

Family medicine reform includes changes in curricula for undergraduate medical studies, and the development of specific training and gradual retraining of existing general practitioners working in both the public and private sectors. Delocalized campuses are being designed to support training of family health teams using the important network of first line facilities. The social responsibilities of medical schools are being strengthened through a focus on health promotion and protection.

Financial and non-financial incentives, including recognition of the specialty of family medicine, are being negotiated between ministries of health, medical schools and the ministry of higher education. Efforts are planned to improve working conditions of health teams working in primary care and to seek more active community participation and empowerment.

REFERENCES

1. Mtiraoui A, Gueddana N. The family and reproductive health program in underprivileged areas in Tunisia; *Actes CICRED Seminar on Reproductive Health, Unmet Needs and Poverty: Issues of Access and Quality of Services,* Bangkok 25–30 November 2002, pp 11.
2. Forum national sur la santé. Rapport de synthèse du groupe de travail sur les déterminants de la santé. 1997. Available from: http://www.hc-sc.gc.ca/hcs-sss/pubs/care-soins/1997-nfoh-fnss-v2/legacy_her itage4_f.html

CHAPTER 33

United Arab Emirates

Haifa Hamad Fares Al Ali and Wadeia Mohammed Al Sharief

Total number of PHC facilities	131
Number of general practitioners working in public PHC facilities	968
Number of certified family physicians working in PHC facilities	382
Average number of family physician graduates/year	25
Number of medical schools	6
Number of family medicine departments	6

INTRODUCTION

The United Arab Emirates (UAE) health-care sector is divided between public and private health-care providers. Public health-care (PHC) services are managed and regulated by the Federal Ministry of Health and Prevention (MoHAP) and local government entities such as the Department of Health Abu Dhabi, the Abu Dhabi Health Services Company (SEHA), and Dubai Health Authority (DHA). The UAE Vision 2021, which is well aligned with United Nations Sustainable Development Goal (SDG) targets, states that "the UAE [will] … invest continually to build world-class health-care infrastructure, expertise and services in order to fulfil citizens' growing needs and expectations".[1] This vision aims to increase the standard of health care through the accreditation of all health facilities by 2021. It also aims to reduce non-communicable diseases (NCD) and increase healthy lifestyles in the community. To reach this vision, a national agenda was developed by the government with measurable indicators. PHC focuses on family medicine as a medical specialty that provides continuous, integrated, and comprehensive health care for individuals and families.

The country has made remarkable progress in all maternal and child health indicators.[2,3] The model of an NCD clinic within PHC provides integrated preventive, treatment, and control care to patients with diabetes, hypertension, dyslipidaemia, chronic pulmonary diseases, and mental illnesses. The school health programme is one of the pioneer PHC programmes that deliver preventive, promotive, and curative services. Smoking cessation counselling services in primary care motivate and support smokers to quit smoking. At present, there are 382 certified family physicians working in the public sector. All newly recruited PHC workers undergo a competency-based programme. 85% of PHC centres are using electronic health records. The government introduced a patient smart portal application through which users can have access to their records. 60% of public primary care centres are accredited by the Joint Commission International Accreditation (JCIA); the target is to reach 100% by 2021.

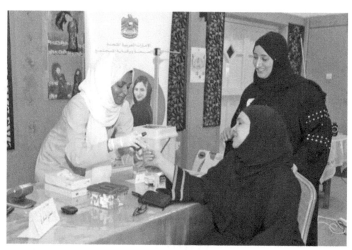

Screening and awareness

KEY CHALLENGES

[1] Workforce development is an area that requires significant and sustainable growth. Only 3% nurses in the country are Emirati and on average 25 family physicians graduate each year. [2] The demographic shift which will double the percentage of Emiratis aged above 60 years by 2032 is posing a big challenge to improving geriatric care in the country. [3] High prevalence of cardiovascular disease, obesity, and diabetes increases the burden on health care. These problems are well recognized by the government and well-structured actions are implemented within the national agenda. [4] Activity around medical research, including primary care-related research, is limited in the UAE. [5] Currently, with the tremendous development in the private health care sector, there is overutilization of certain types of services, which increases costs and reduces efficiency.

WAY FORWARD

The Primary Care Medical Home (PCMH), or Baytona Al Tebbi, is a system improvement project adapted by ambulatory health services in the Abu Dhabi Health Services Company (SEHA); it is a model of care based on family medicine principles. The model is based on enhanced access, personal providers and patient engagement and self-management. The patient registered to any primary care centre will consider the centre his or her medical home. The primary care physician, as the primary care provider (PCP), will be accountable for meeting that patient's current and future needs. Mobile clinics have been introduced and deployed to serve remote areas of Abu Dhabi Emirate that have difficulty in accessing health-care facilities, and to bring health-care services to users at public events, work sites, and schools. In 2016, the MoHAP also introduced the mobile health clinic. An elderly care unit, consisting of a multidisciplinary team with a geriatrician, family medicine physician, community medicine physician, physiatrist, physiotherapist, nurses, social worker, and dietitian, has been introduced.

REFERENCES

1. *UAE Vision 2021, National Agenda.* Available from: https://www.vision2021.ae/en [Accessed: 9 January 2019].
2. UAE Demographics Profile 2017. Available from: https://www.indexmundi.com/united_arab_emirates/demographics_profile.html [Accessed: 9 January 2019].
3. World Health Organization. *WHO Vaccine-Preventable Diseases: Monitoring System. 2018 Global Summary.* Available from: http://apps.who.int/immunization_monitoring/globalsummary/countries?countrycriteria%5Bcountry%5D%5B%5D=ARE&commit=OK [Accessed: 9 January 2019].

CHAPTER 34

Yemen

Ali Al-Mudhwahi

Total number of PHC facilities	Total HFs: 4602
	Others: 3
Number of general practitioners working in public PHC facilities	2389
Number of certified family physicians working in PHC facilities	3
Average number of family physician graduates/year	6
Number of medical schools	9
Number of family medicine departments	3

Hospitals: 255, HCs: 1055, HUs: 3289
HF, health facility; HC, health centre; HU, health unit; PHC, primary health care

INTRODUCTION

The ongoing war in Yemen has left 18.8 million people in need of humanitarian assistance and placed an overwhelming strain on the country's health system at a time when it is most needed. Approximately 7 million people are in dire need of food, and levels of malnutrition are on the rise, leaving the country on the brink of famine. Almost 462,000 children suffer from severe acute malnutrition with a risk of life-threatening complications. Less than 45% of health facilities are fully functioning: at least 274 of them have been damaged or destroyed during the current conflict, which started in March 2015.[1] Health-care workers have been forced to relocate and the ones still working do not receive their salaries regularly.

Supported by the Global Alliance for Vaccines, the Ministry of Public Health and Population (MoPHP) initiated an integrated approach in its delivery of basic health services, using fixed facilities and outreach sessions. The district health system represented the basis on which the model of integration was developed. The under-five mortality rate dropped by nearly 50% from 102 in 2003, to 51 in 2013; the maternal mortality ratio dropped from 365 to 148 during the same period. Recently, the MoPHP, with the support of the WHO, has started to implement the Minimum Service Package. Between 2006–2010, the MoPHP developed training manuals, guidelines and policy on integrated services.

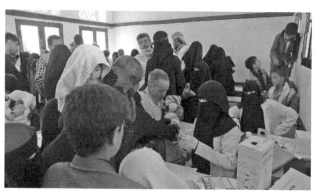

Immunization campaign

The possibility of achieving universal health coverage is limited by the inaccessibility of health care and financial barriers[2]. The essential drug list was last updated in 2014 and contains 437 items. Yemen was ranked as number 160 out of 188 countries in the Human Development Index. Yemen ranks lowest of the 155 countries listed in the Gender Inequality Index. Numbers of qualified health personnel in rural areas are inadequate, and the war has forced many of them to flee their homes.

KEY CHALLENGES

The most common causes of death are lower respiratory tract infection (28%), ischemic heart disease (9.5%), stroke (6.8%), preterm birth complications (6.6%) and road injury (3.8).[3] Despite efforts to reduce high maternal and under-five mortality rates, malnutrition continues to be a major health problem. High levels of stunting, underweight, and wasting were already documented in the Family Health Survey of 2003, before the war.[4] Considering the overwhelming challenges facing the country, family practice is currently at a crossroads in terms of its implementation. Security challenges and growing demands for trauma care have weakened the ability of family practice to deliver on its promises. Health-care providers are unable to optimally perform their duties due to the ongoing political and economic crises.

WAY FORWARD

As part of strengthening the national health system, the MoPHP adopted a family-centred care approach. It established a family health general directorate, led by a Deputy Minister, which works towards an integrated approach to health-care decision making within the PHC sector. Before March 2015, the family health department of the MoPHP had been successful in leading integrated primary health-care interventions through PHC facilities and outreach activities. The focus on core public health programmes was well demonstrated at the local level, through capacity building programmes that enhanced the provision of basic health services. The integrated approach of primary health-care services resulted in significant improvements in maternal and child health. This improvement has been set back since the start of the war in March 2015. The MoPHP views the private sector as a potential partner for development, which can be contracted to provide coverage in areas the public sector cannot, especially for immunization and reproductive health services.

REFERENCES

1. WHO, *Health Resources Availability Mapping System* (HeRAMS), Yemen, 2017.
2. MoPHP. Yemen. *NHS 2010–2025*. 2010. Available from: http://www.nationalplanni ngcycles.org/sites/default/files/planning_cycle_repository/yemen/nat_health_strategy_-_yemen_en g.pdf [Accessed 24 April 2018].
3. *The Health Cluster Response Strategy to Yemen's Crisis for 2015–2016*, Yemen, October 2015.
4. MoPHP, Yemen. *Family Health Survey, Yemen, 2003*.

ممارسة طب الأسرة
في إقليم شرق المتوسط

احتفالاً بيوم الصحة العالمي 2019

طب الأسرة للمنظمة العالمية لأطباء الأسرة

نبذة عن السلسلة

سلسلة طب الأسرة للمنظمة العالمية لأطباء الأسرة هي مجموعة كتب من تأليف خبراء وممارسي طب الأسرة من شتى أنحاء العالم، بالتعاون مع المنظمة العالمية لأطباء الأسرة.

والمنظمة العالمية لأطباء الأسرة هي منظمة غير ربحية أنشأتها في عام 1972 منظماتٌ أعضاء في 18 بلداً، وتضم الآن 118 منظمةً عضواً في 131 بلداً وإقليماً، ويبلغ مجموع أعضائها نحو 500 ألف طبيب أسرة، وأكثر من 90 في المائة من سكان العالم.

صحة اللاجئين والمهاجرين
من منظور الرعاية الصحية الأولية
برناديت كومار، وإسبرنزا دياز

الرعاية الصحية الأولية في أنحاء العالم
توصيات بشأن السياسة الدولية والتنمية
كريس فان ويل، وأماندا هاو

ممارسة طب الأسرة في إقليم شرق المتوسط
التغطية الصحية الشاملة والرعاية الأولية الجيدة
حسن صلاح، ومايكل كيد

كل طبيب
أطباء بصحة أفضل = مرضى بصحة أوفر
ليان رو، ومايكل كيد

كيفية إجراء بحوث الرعاية الأولية
فيليسيتي جودير-سميث، وبوب ماش

طب الأسرة
الورقات البحثيَّة الكلاسيكية
مايكل كيد، وإيونا هيث، وأماندا هاو

وجهات نظر دولية بشأن بحوث الرعاية الأولية
فيليسيتي غودير سميث، وبوب ماش

مساهمة طب الأسرة في تحسين النُظُم الصحية
دليل من المنظمة العالمية لأطباء الأسرة
مايكل كيد

ممارسة طب الأسرة
في إقليم شرق المتوسط

الرعاية الصحية الأولية
من أجل التغطية الصحية الشاملة

تحرير:

حسن صلاح ● مايكل كيد ● أحمد منديل

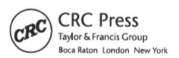

CRC Press
Taylor & Francis Group
Boca Raton London New York

CRC Press is an imprint of the
Taylor & Francis Group, an **informa** business

CRC Press

Taylor & Francis Group

6000 Broken Sound Parkway NW, Suite 300

Boca Raton, FL 33487-2742

نُهدي هذه الدراسة الأحادية إلى شعوب الدول الأعضاء في إقليم شرق المتوسط،

وإلى القوى العاملة في مجال الرعاية الصحية في الإقليم،

وإلى النساء والرجال الذين كرّسوا حياتهم لتقديم رعاية صحية أولية عالية الجودة

للشعوب والمجتمعات التي يخدمونها.

تعد ممارسة طب الأسرة أفضل طريقة لتقديم خدمات صحية متكاملة على مستوى الرعاية الصحية الأولية. فمن خلال التركيز على تعزيز الصحة والوقاية من الأمراض، تساعد ممارسة طب الأسرة على النَّأي بالناس عن المستشفيات، حيث تكون التكاليف أكبر وغالباً ما تكون النتائج أسوأ. إن الالتزام السياسي القوي أساسي لتحسين إتاحة الخدمات الصحية والتغطية بها ومقبوليتها وجودتها، ولضمان استمرارية الرعاية.

الدكتور تيدروس أدهانوم غيبريسوس
المدير العام لمنظمة الصحة العالمية

المحتويات

تمهيد

لقد وقع الاختيار على الرعاية الصحية الأولية لتكون محور يوم الصحة العالمي لعام 2019. ويأتي يوم الصحة العالمي هذا العام في منتصف الفترة الفاصلة بين المؤتمر العالمي للرعاية الصحية الأولية لعام 2018 الذي عُقد في مدينة أستانا، والاجتماع الرفيع المستوى للجمعية العامة للأمم المتحدة بشأن التغطية الصحية الشاملة الذي سيُعقد في نيويورك في أيلول/سبتمبر 2019. ويتيح هذا اليوم فرصة عظيمة لمنظمة الصحة العالمية لكي تكرر وتعزز دعوتنا إلى توفير الصحة للجميع وبالجميع – مع التركيز على الدور الحاسم للرعاية الصحية الأولية في تحقيق التغطية الصحية الشاملة. وتتناول فصول هذه الدراسة الأحادية كلاً من الخبرات القُطرية والأبعاد الرئيسية التي تؤثر في التغطية الصحية الشاملة، ويجب أن تشمل: قدرات النُّظُم بأكملها، ونماذج التمويل، والقوى العاملة والتدريب، والرعاية المتكاملة القائمة على الاحتياجات. وينصب التركيز على كلٍّ من المجالات الذاتية والموضوعية – ما يريده المرضى، وكيف يمكن زيادة أعمارهم وفرصهم إلى أقصى حدٍّ من خلال التدخلات الصحية والرعاية الصحية الفعالة المُيَسَّرة، وكيفية تلبية احتياجات السكان. ويُمعن النظر أيضاً في القوى العاملة الصحية الحديثة، مع الاستعانة على نحو مناسب بالفرق المتعددة التخصصات والتقنيات المعلوماتية الحديثة.

ومن أكثر الأمور المستحدثة في هذه الدراسة الأحادية هو تركيزها على طب الأسرة وممارسته – وهو تخصصٌ جديد بالنسبة للكثيرين، ونهجٌ ما زال يجري تطبيقه في أنحاء كثيرة من الإقليم. وعلى الصعيد العالمي، شهدت السنوات الخمسون الماضية توجُّهَ جميع الأطباء إلى تلقي تدريب تخصصي. ويعني ذلك، فيما يخص الرعاية الصحية الأولية، تدريب أطباء عامّين يستطيعون الجمع بين التشخيص والتثقيف الصحي والعلاج والرعاية المستمرة للمرضى في مختلف المراحل العمرية ولشتى المشاكل الصحية. وقد كان، ولا يزال، إقليم شرق المتوسط مُبدِعاً في محاولة الارتقاء بمستوى "الأطباء العامّين" من أجل تلبية احتياجات وفرص مواطني القرن الحادي والعشرين، وقد وضع الإقليم في اعتباره البيّنات المتزايدة التي تشير إلى أن أطباء الأسرة الذين يتلقون تدريباً تخصصياً بعد التخرج يوفرون تكاليف كبيرة لأي نظام صحي؛ لأنهم يستخدمون مهاراتهم في التشخيص المبكر، ويتعاملون مع المشاكل المتعددة في وقت واحد، ويدعمون كلًّا من فرقهم ومرضاهم للعمل معاً على تحقيق أقصى قدر ممكن من المكاسب الصحية. فالخبرة الطبية باهظة الثمن، واستخدامها على أفضل وجه جانب رئيسي من جوانب التغطية الصحية العالية الجودة الميسورة التكلفة. وأما غير الملِمّين بممارسة طب الأسرة، فإن هذه الدراسة الأحادية تقدم لهم رؤى رئيسية حول كيفية دمج البلدان لهذه القوى العاملة الجديدة في نظمها الصحية، وتوضح كيف يمكن لها أن تضيف قيمة.

ولا أحد، بطبيعة الحال، يحقق أي شيء بمفرده. فالتغطية الصحية الشاملة الفعالة تحتاج إلى تمويل مناسب، وبنية تحتية، وإجراءات بشأن أسباب اعتلال الصحة، فضلاً عن قوة عاملة قوية. ويعتمد الأثر الذي يتركه أطباء الأسرة على النظام الذي يعملون تحت مظلته، والظروف التي يعملون فيها، والفريق الذي يعملون معه. ومن دواعي سرور منظمة الصحة العالمية والمنظمة العالمية لأطباء الأسرة أن تَرَيَا احتفاء هذه الدراسة الأحادية بعمل الكثيرين في إقليم شرق المتوسط، ونأمل أن تسهم هذه الدراسة الأحادية في الرعاية الصحية لشعوب الإقليم ورفاهيتهم في المستقبل. شكراً جزيلاً لكل مَن شارك فيها.

الدكتور أحمد بن سالم المنظري
مدير منظمة الصحة العالمية
لإقليم شرق المتوسط

الأستاذ دونالد لي
رئيس المنظمة العالمية لأطباء الأسرة

مقدمة

إننا نحتفل بيوم الصحة العالمي تحت شعار "الرعاية الصحية الأولية من أجل تحقيق التغطية الصحية الشاملة" بنشر هذه الدراسة الأحادية الخاصة بإقليم شرق المتوسط. وقد اجتمع قادة العالم يومي 25 و26 تشرين الأول/أكتوبر 2018 لتجديد التزامهم بتعزيز الرعاية الصحية الأولية من أجل تحقيق التغطية الصحية الشاملة وأهداف التنمية المستدامة. ويتجسد ذلك الالتزام في إعلان جديد يؤكد الحاجةَ إلى تحديث خدمات الرعاية الصحية الأولية، ومجابهة التحديات الحالية والمستقبلية التي تواجه النُظُم الصحية، مع الحفاظ في الوقت ذاته على القيم الأساسية والمبادئ الواردة في إعلان ألما-آتا الأصلي الصادر في عام 1978.

والتغطية الصحية الشاملة تعني أن يستطيع جميع الناس والمجتمعات المحلية الحصول على الخدمات الصحية التي يحتاجون إليها، سواء أكانت خدمات تعزيزية أم وقائية أم علاجية أم تأهيلية أم ملطّفة، وأن تكون هذه الخدمات على درجة كافية من الجودة بما يضمن فاعليتها، على ألّا يتعرضوا لضائقة مالية من جراء استفادتهم من تلك الخدمات. وتتطلب مسيرتنا صوْب تحقيق التغطية الصحية الشاملة تقوية النُظم الصحية، بما في ذلك التصدي للمُحدِّدات الاجتماعية والبيئية للصحة على نحو فعّال عبر العمل المشترك بين القطاعات. وتُمثل الحماية الصحية الاجتماعية والإنصاف اعتبارين رئيسيَين في التغطية الصحية الشاملة.

ويفتقر نصف سكان العالم إلى إمكانية الحصول على الخدمات الصحية الأساسية، وينطبق ذلك بالتأكيد على جزء كبير من سكان إقليم شرق المتوسط. وكما قال الدكتور تيدروس، المدير العام لمنظمة الصحة العالمية: "إن تحقيق التغطية الصحية الشاملة يمثِّل تحدياً سياسياً أكثر من كونه تحدياً اقتصادياً". ومن خلال اعتماد خطة التنمية المستدامة لعام 2030، تعهدت دول العالم بتحقيق التغطية الصحية الشاملة بحلول عام 2030، مما يعني أنه يوجد بالفعل التزام عالمي. وقد حان الآن وقت تحويل هذا الالتزام العالمي إلى عمل وطني. وتشير تقديرات البنك الدولي إلى أنه يمكن تلبية 90% من جميع الاحتياجات الصحية على مستوى الرعاية الصحية الأولية.[1] كما أن الاستثمار في بناء خدمات الرعاية الصحية الأولية الجيدة والمُنصفة التي يَسهل الحصول عليها يُعدّ الخطوةَ العملية الأولى الأكثر كفاءةً وفاعليةً للبلدان التي تعمل على تحقيق التغطية الصحية الشاملة.

وفي أيار/مايو 2016، اعتمدت جمعية الصحة العالمية التاسعة والستون، بموجب القرار WHA 69.24، إطار عمل لتعزيز الخدمات الصحية المتكاملة التي تُركِّز على الناس. وفي هذا القرار، حثَّت جمعية الصحة العالمية الدول الأعضاء على أن تُنفِّذ هذا الإطار، حسب مقتضى الحال. وأن تجعل نُظُم الرعاية الصحية أكثر استجابة لاحتياجات الناس. وتَبِع ذلك، في تشرين الأول/أكتوبر 2016، اعتماد القرار EM/RC63/R.2 بشأن توسيع نطاق ممارسة طب الأسْرة: التقدم المُحرز من أجل تحقيق التغطية الصحية الشاملة. وفي هذا القرار، حثَّت اللجنة الإقليمية الدول الأعضاء على إدراج نهج ممارسة طب الأسْرة في خدمات الرعاية الصحية الأولية باعتباره استراتيجية جامعة للمُضي قُدُماً صوْب تحقيق التغطية الصحية الشاملة.

ويمكن تعريف ممارسة طب الأسْرة بأنها خدمات الرعاية الصحية التي يُقدِّمها طبيب الأسْرة وفريقه، وتتميز بأنها خدمات شاملة ومُجتمعية المنحى ومستمرة ومُنسَّقة وتعاونية وشخصية وأسرية حسب احتياجات الفرد وأسرته في جميع المراحل العمرية.

وهناك التزام سياسي متزايد لدى بلدان إقليم شرق المتوسط باعتماد نهج ممارسة طب الأسْرة من أجل تحسين مستوى تقديم الخدمات. وعلى الرغم من هذا الالتزام، فلا تزال ممارسة طب الأسْرة تواجه تحديات هائلة في معظم الدول الأعضاء في الإقليم، منها قصور البنى التحتية للمرافق الصحية، وتدنّي الوعي المجتمعي، وعدم كفاية القدرات التقنية اللازمة للتوسع في هذا النهج.

---

[1] Doherty G and Govender R, 'The cost effectiveness of primary care services in developing countries: A review of international literature', Working Paper No. 37, Disease Control Priorities Project, World Bank, WHO and Fogarty International Centre of the U.S. National Institutes of Health, 2004, https://www.researchgate.net/publication/242783643_The_Cost-Effectiveness_of_Primary_Care_Services_in_Developing_Countries_A_Review_of_the_International_Literature Henceforth 'World Bank Report'.

ويعني نقص عدد أطباء الأسرة المؤهلين أن 93% من المرافق الصحية يديرها أطباء لم يتلقوا تدريباً تخصصياً بعد التخرج. وتسهم الصورة السيئة للعديد من الخدمات الصحية التي يقدمها القطاع العام في قلة الاستفادة من تلك الخدمات. ويُضاعف غيابُ نُظُم الإحالة الفعالة وشبكات المستشفيات الجيدة من تدني جودة الخدمات وكفاءتها.

وهناك تحديات كبيرة ماثلة أمام ضمان المشاركة الفعالة للقطاع الصحي الخاص ومساهمته في التحرك صوب تحقيق الأهداف الصحية العامة. وينشط القطاع الصحي الخاص نشاطاً ملحوظاً فيما يتعلق بتقديم خدمات الرعاية بالعيادات الخارجية داخل إقليم شرق المتوسط. فيقدم العاملون في القطاع الصحي الخاص في الإقليم ما يصل إلى 70% من خدمات العيادات الخارجية. وينبغي أن يؤخذ ذلك في الاعتبار عند وضع الاستراتيجيات الرامية إلى تعزيز الرعاية الصحية الأولية واستحداث ممارسة طب الأسرة. وقد نما القطاع الصحي الخاص بالقدر الأدنى من التوجيه والدعم على مستوى السياسات، بل يَندُر أن يكون جزءاً من عمليات تخطيط القطاع الصحي التي تجريها الحكومات. وقد برز دور القطاع الخاص في العديد من البلدان، نتيجة قصور الخدمات الصحية التي يقدمها القطاع العام وعدم ارتقاء أدائها إلى المستوى المأمول. وتُعد المشاركة الفعالة مع القطاع الصحي الخاص لتقديم الخدمات عبر نهُج ممارسة طب الأسرة عنصراً مهماً من أجل تحقيق التغطية الصحية الشاملة.

وهذه الدراسة الأحادية نتاج جهد تعاوني بين منظمة الصحة العالمية والمنظمة العالمية لأطباء الأسرة. وهي أول مسعى من هذا القبيل في إقليم شرق المتوسط. وتضم 34 فصلاً، منها فصول خاصة بالإقليم تسلط الضوء على العديد من موضوعات السياسات ذات الصلة بإقليم شرق المتوسط وكيفية معالجتها في شتى أنحاء الإقليم، وفصول تلخص الوضع الحالي لممارسة طب الأسرة في كل بلد من البلدان الاثنين والعشرين لإقليم شرق المتوسط. ويمثل المؤلفون طائفة واسعة من الخبراء العالميين والإقليميين والوطنيين في مجال ممارسة طب الأسرة. وتتناول الفصول الخاصة بالبلدان الرعاية الصحية الأولية وتطوير ممارسة طب الأسرة في كل بلد، مع التركيز على التحديات والنجاحات والدروس المستفادة.

وهذه الدراسة الأحادية مُوجَّهة إلى راسمي السياسات، والمهنيين الصحيين، والطلاب والمُعلمين في مجال الصحة. وتُناقش سُبُل تطوير الرعاية الصحية الأولية وتحسينها في البلدان ذات الدخل المرتفع والمتوسط والمنخفض، وكذلك في البلدان التي تشهد حالات طوارئ.

حسن صلاح (محرر)، ومايكل كيد (محرر)،
وظفر ميرزا (مدير تطوير النُظُم الصحية،
المكتب الإقليمي لمنظمة الصحة العالمية لشرق المتوسط)
آذار/مارس 2019

شكر وتقدير

وُلدت فكرة الكتاب الذي أعقبته هذه الدراسة الأحادية أثناء المناقشات التي جرت بين منظمة الصحة العالمية والمنظمة العالمية لأطباء الأسرة لطب الأسرة خلال المؤتمر الرابع في إقليم شرق المتوسط الذي عقدته المنظمة العالمية لأطباء الأسرة في آذار/مارس 2017 في أبو ظبي بالإمارات العربية المتحدة. وهذا هو أول جهد تعاوني كبير بين المنظمتين في هذا الإقليم.

ونود أن نعرب عن تقديرنا للعمل المتميز والضخم الذي أنجزه تسعون مؤلفاً ومؤلفاً مشاركاً، الذين أسهموا في كتابة 34 فصلاً في هذه الدراسة الأحادية، وهم يمثلون مجموعة ذائعة الصيت من خبراء الرعاية الصحية الأولية على الصعيد الوطني والإقليمي والعالمي، الذين تطوعوا بوقتهم وعلمهم من أجل هذا العمل. لقد سعِدنا بالعمل معهم، ونتطلع إلى بدء المرحلة التالية من إعداد الإصدار الثاني من الدراسة، المُقرر صدوره في تشرين الأول/أكتوبر 2020.

ونتوجه بالشكر إلى العاملين في قسم تطوير النظم الصحية بالمكتب الإقليمي لمنظمة الصحة العالمية لشرق المتوسط الذين شاركوا في مراجعة الفصول القُطرية الاثنين والعشرين: الدكتور عدي النصيرات، والدكتور إلكر داستن، والدكتور أدهم إسماعيل، والدكتور منذر لطيف، والدكتورة أروى عويس، والدكتور حميد رافاقي، والدكتور جوهر واجد.

كذلك نتوجه بالشكر إلى السيد جي بينيه، والسيد إدريس أبو الحسين، وفريق النشر ودعم الموقع الإلكتروني بالمكتب الإقليمي للمنظمة على مراجعة الفصول العربية والفرنسية لهذه الدراسة الأحادية، ونشكر أيضاً المحررين المحترفين، والسيدة أليس جرينجر جاسر، والسيدة سوزي بالابان، والسيدة ليزلي وايتنج.

ونتوجه بشكر خاص إلى السيد حاتم عادل الخضري، مدير قسم الشؤون الإدارية والمالية في المكتب الإقليمي للمنظمة، وإلى السيد كينيث تشارلز بيرسي من قسم الشؤون القانونية في المقر الرئيسي للمنظمة، على الانتهاء من الإجراءات التعاقدية المتشعبة بين تايلور آند فرانسيس/سي آر سي برس، ومنظمة الصحة العالمية، والمنظمة العالمية لأطباء الأسرة.

ونشكر الدكتور جارث مانينغ، الرئيس التنفيذي للمنظمة العالمية لأطباء الأسرة، على دعمه المستمر لهذا التعاون وغيره من أوجه التعاون الكثيرة بين منظمته ومنظمة الصحة العالمية.

ونتوجه بالشكر إلى الحكومة اليابانية على دعمها المالي لمنظمة الصحة العالمية من أجل تحقيق التغطية الصحية الشاملة. ونعرب عن بالغ تقديرنا للشراكة القائمة بين الاتحاد الأوروبي ولوكسمبرج ومنظمة الصحة العالمية بشأن التغطية الصحية الشاملة على تمويلها السخي، بغرض الدعم الجزئي لهذا المنشور الصادر عن المكتب الإقليمي لمنظمة الصحة العالمية لشرق المتوسط.

وختاماً، نتوجه بالشكر إلى فريق تايلور آند فرانسيس/سي آر سي برس على ما قدموه من دعم كبير طوال عملية إعداد هذه الدراسة الأحادية ونشرها.

التوجُّه العالمي نحو خدمات صحية متكاملة محورها الناس: دور ممارسة طب الأسرة
شانون باركلي، هرنان مونتينيجرو، آن-ليز جيسيت، نوريا تورو بولانكو، ستيفاني نجو، إد كيلي

رغم أوجه التقدم الكبير الذي أُحرز في الصحة ومتوسط العمر المتوقع في السنوات الأخيرة، كانت أوجه التحسُّن متفاوتة فيما بين البلدان وداخل البلد الواحد. وإضافةً إلى ذلك، ما فتئت تظهر تحديات صحية جديدة تتعلق بالتحولات السكانية والوبائية. إذ يواجه سكان العالم التوسّع الحضري، والهجرة، والشيخوخة، والميل نحو أنماط الحياة غير الصحية في كل أنحاء العالم، والعبء المزدوج للأمراض السارية وغير السارية، والحالات المرضية المتعددة، وزيادة أوبئة الأمراض، وحالات الطوارئ المعقدة، علاوة على أن المشاركة الاجتماعية والتوقعات في ازدياد طوال الوقت.

ولأن النظم الصحية لمعظم البلدان قد صُمِّمت لمعالجة مشاكل الماضي الصحية، فإن هذه النظم لا تصلح للتصدي لتحديات القرن الحادي والعشرين. وتشير التقديرات الحالية إلى أن نصف سكان العالم على الأقل لا يزالون يفتقرون إلى الخدمات الصحية الأساسية.[1] وبالإضافة إلى عدم كفاية الاستجابة للعوائق المالية والجغرافية، تزداد صعوبة الحصول على هذه الخدمات في البلدان التي لا تزال تواجه مشاكل في ضمان توفير المستلزمات الأساسية للنظام الصحي، ومنها القوى العاملة الصحية الكافية والأدوية الأساسية. ولا تزال التغطية بالخدمات الأساسية (مثل الرعاية السابقة للولادة ووجود قابلات ماهرات عند الولادة) منخفضةً في كثير من البلدان، حتى في الحالات المرضية ذات الأولوية القصوى مثل صحة الأمهات والأطفال.[2]

وإذا وُجدت الرعاية، فإنها في الغالب تكون مُجزَّأة أو رديئة الجودة. وتتسم استمرارية الرعاية بالضعف في كثير من الحالات الصحية، وهي بالغة الأهمية في حالة الأمراض المزمنة. ويؤدي تجزؤ خدمات الرعاية وسوء تنظيمها، بسبب ضعف نُظُم الإحالة، إلى نتائج أسوأ وتكلفة أكبر. كما أن التركيز على نماذج الرعاية العلاجية «المنعزلة» المستقلة بذاتها والتي تُقدَّم في المستشفيات وتقوم على علاج الأمراض، بدلاً من التركيز بشكل ملائم على الرعاية الصحية الأولية، يزيد من إضعاف قدرة النظم الصحية على تقديم رعاية شاملة ومنصفة وفائقة الجودة ومستدامة مالياً. ويمكن لمنصات تقديم الخدمات الموازية أن تسهم بقدر أكبر في التجزؤ، بسبب سعي الناس إلى الحصول على الرعاية في كلا القطاعين العام والخاص.

وفي هذا السياق، اعتمدت البلدان في عام 2015 أهداف التنمية المستدامة، ومنها الهدف الثالث الخاص بالصحة: ضمان تمتع الجميع بأنماط عيش صحية وبالرفاهية في جميع الأعمار.[3] وتُعدُّ الغاية الثامنة للهدف الثالث من أهداف التنمية المستدامة – تحقيق التغطية الصحية الشاملة، بما في ذلك إتاحة خدمات الرعاية الصحية الأساسية الجيدة – غاية أساسية لبلوغ هدف الصحة للجميع. وتعني التغطية الصحية الشاملة حصول جميع الأفراد والمجتمعات على الخدمات الصحية التي يحتاجون إليها دون التعرض لضائقة مالية. ولكي تكون خدمات التغطية الصحية الشاملة فعالة ويكون تمويل الخدمات مستداماً، لا بد من إجراء تغيير أساسي في طريقة تنظيم الخدمات وتقديمها.

ويشمل ذلك إعادة توجيه الخدمات الصحية لضمان توفير الرعاية في الموقع الأكثر ملاءمة وفعالية من حيث التكلفة، مع تحقيق التوازن الصحيح بين الرعاية الخارجية والداخلية وتعزيز تنسيق الرعاية عبر المواقع. وينبغي أن تتمحور الخدمات الصحية حول الاحتياجات والتوقعات الشاملة للأشخاص والمجتمعات المحلية، مع تمكينهم من الاضطلاع بدور أنشط في صحتهم ونظامهم الصحي.

ويرتبط التوجُّه نحو الرعاية الصحية الأولية داخل النظم الصحية بتحقيق أفضل مخرجات تكون فيها الرعاية متاحة ومنصفة وفعالة وآمنة ومتمحورة حول الناس – ومن ثمَّ فهو ضروري لتحقيق أهداف التغطية الفعالة. كما أن التوجُّه نحو الرعاية الصحية الأولية فعال من حيث التكاليف، مما يعزز استدامة تمويل النظام الصحي ويسمح بالتحقيق التدريجي للتغطية الصحية الشاملة. كما ترتبط الرعاية الصحية الأولية بارتفاع مستويات القدرة على الاستجابة، مع تركيزها على رعاية جميع الأشخاص والتنسيق والاستمرارية.[4]

وقد حددت البحوث التي أُجريت على مدار العقود الماضية الخصائص المشتركة بين نظم الرعاية الأولية ذات الأداء الرفيع، أيْ تلك الصفات التي يجب أن تضمن أن الرعاية الأولية تؤدي وظيفتها الحيوية. وتؤثر هذه الخصائص في مدى إتاحة الرعاية الأولية وإنصافها وفعاليتها من حيث التكاليف ومأمونيتها وكفاءتها، وتتمثل فيما يلي: تصدُّر مراحل التواصل، التمحور حول الناس، الاستمرارية، الشمول، التنسيق، التوجه نحو الأسرة والمجتمع، بالإضافة إلى احتلال مكانة محورية في نهج ممارسة طب الأسرة.[5]

ونظراً إلى أهميتها الأساسية في النظم الصحية، لم يخلُ جدول أعمال السياسات قط من الرعاية الأولية، ولكنها لا تزال في بلدان كثيرة لا تحظى بالاهتمام أو الموارد أو الدعم اللازم للاضطلاع بدورها الجوهري. ونتيجة لذلك، لا تتحقق في الغالب جميع إمكانيات الرعاية الأولية. فلكي تؤدي الرعاية الأولية دورها الحاسم في تلبية الاحتياجات الصحية المستقبلية، يجب أن تتصدى الإصلاحات للدعم الهيكلي والمالي فضلاً عن إعادة توجيه نماذج الرعاية الصحية للوفاء بالمتطلبات الصحية الحالية.

وتسمح ممارسة طب الأسرة بتقديم رعاية صحية أولية رفيعة الأداء. كما أن تحويل النظم الصحية لتكون أكثر تكاملاً وتركيزاً على الناس، بما في ذلك التأكيد المتجدد على الرعاية الصحية الأولية، يمكن أن يذلل ما يوجد حالياً من تحديات سكانية ووبائية وصعوبات تتعلق بالنظم الصحية.

المراجع

1. World Health Organization and the International Bank for Reconstruction and Development / The World Bank. Tracking Universal Health Coverage: 2017 Global Monitoring Report. Geneva : World Health Organization, 2017.
2. Countdown to 2015: maternal, newborn and child survival. Country Profiles. [على الإنترنت] [جرى الاطلاع عليه في: 22 كانون الثاني/يناير 2018].
3. United Nations. Sustainable Development Goals: 17 Goals to Transform our World. [على الإنترنت] [جرى الاطلاع عليه في: 22 كانون الثاني/يناير 2018]. http://www.un.org/sustainabledevelopment/health/.
4. World Health Organization. People-centred and integrated health services: a review of the evidence. Geneva : WHO Press, 2015. WHO/HIS/SDS/2015.7.
5. Starfield B, Shi L, Macinko J. Contribution of primary care to health systems and health. Millbank Quarterly, 2005; 83: 457-502.

توسيع نطاق ممارسة طب الأسرة: التقدم صوب تحقيق التغطية الصحية الشاملة في إقليم شرق المتوسط
ظفر ميرزا، محمد أسائي أردكاني، حسن صلاح

اعتمدت الدورة التاسعة والستون لجمعية الصحة العالمية، التي عُقدت في أيار/مايو 2016، قرار جمعية الصحة العالمية رقم 69-24 بشأن "تعزيز الخدمات الصحية المتكاملة التي تُركِّز على الناس". وفي هذا القرار حثَّت جمعية الصحة العالمية الدولَ الأعضاء على أن تُنفِّذ إطار العمل، حسب مقتضى الحال، وأن تجعل نُظم الرعاية الصحية أكثر استجابة لاحتياجات الناس. وتُطبَّق هذه الاستراتيجية في المكتب الإقليمي لمنظمة الصحة العالمية لشرق المتوسط على مستوى خدمة الرعاية الأولية من خلال برنامج ممارسة طب الأسرة. واعتمدت اللجنة الإقليمية لشرق المتوسط، في دورتها الثالثة والستين التي عُقدت في تشرين الأول/أكتوبر 2016، قرار البند 4(أ) من جدول الأعمال "توسيع نطاق طب الأسرة: التقدُّم المُحرَز من أجل تحقيق التغطية الصحية الشاملة". وحثَّ هذا القرار الدول الأعضاء على دمج نهج ممارسة طب الأسرة في خدمات الرعاية الصحية الأولية باعتباره استراتيجية جامعة للمُضي قُدُماً صَوُب تحقيق التغطية الصحية الشاملة.

ويمكن تعريف ممارسة طب الأسرة بأنها خدمات الرعاية الصحية التي يُقدِّمها طبيب الأسرة وأعضاء فريقه، وتتميز بأنها خدمات شاملة ومُجتمعية المنحى ومستمرة ومُنسَّقة وتعاونية وشخصية وأسرية حسب احتياجات الفرد وأسرته في جميع المراحل العمرية. وتُعتبر ممارسة طب الأسرة، بوصفها البوابة الأولى للحصول على الخدمة الصحية، عنصراً أساسياً في تقديم خدمات صحية فعالة وتحسين الصحة من خلال سبل شاملة تضمن استمرارية الرعاية. ويمكن لممارسة طب الأسرة أن تلبي معظم احتياجات الأفراد والأسر والمجتمعات المحلية فيما يخص الصحة والرعاية الصحية.[1]

وغالباً ما يُستخدم مصطلحا "ممارسة طب الأسرة" و"طب الأسرة" مترادفين في المؤلفات والدراسات. ويُعرَّف "طب الأسرة" بأنه تخصص طبي يُعنى بتوفير رعاية شاملة للأفراد والأُسر، ويجمع بين العلوم الطبية الحيوية والسلوكية والاجتماعية. ولأنه مبحث طبي أكاديمي، فإنه يتضمن خدمات الرعاية الصحية الشاملة والتعليم والبحوث.[2]

ويتطلب نطاق الخدمات المُقدَّمة من خلال ممارسة طب الأسرة فريقاً متعدد التخصصات، ويركز جوهر ممارسة طب الأسرة على نهج العمل الجماعي في تقديم الخدمات. وقد يختلف تشكيل الفريق المُقدِّم للخدمات من بلد إلى آخر حسب حزمة الخدمات والهياكل والموارد وتوفر الموارد البشرية، ولكن يجب أن يتضمن الفريق طبيب أسرة وممرضة على الأقل.

وتشير الأدلة إلى أن فريق طب الأسرة المُدرَّب تدريباً جيداً يُسهم في تحسين الحصول على رعاية جيدة.[3] ورغم أن طبيب الأسرة والممرضة هما عِمادا ممارسة طب الأسرة، فهناك نقص في جميع أنحاء العالم في أطباء الأسرة، ويتفاقم هذا النقص في إقليم شرق المتوسط.

وإلى جانب تحسين القدرات التدريبية، ينبغي مراعاة ديناميكيات سوق العمل عند اجتذاب العاملين الصحيين واستبقائهم للعمل في مواقع ممارسة طب الأسرة. وتواجه معظم بلدان إقليم شرق المتوسط تحديات تتعلق بالقوى العاملة في مواقع الرعاية الصحية الأولية، لا سيما في المناطق الريفية والنائية. ولذلك ينبغي تقديم حوافز كافية لتشجيع الأطباء على التخصص في طب الأسرة، وكذلك لتشجيع غيرهم من المهنيين على الانضمام إلى فريق ممارسة طب الأسرة. وهذه الحوافز، التي قد تكون حوافز مالية وغير مالية، وكذلك حوافز مهنية وشخصية، يجب أن يكون هدفها تلبية احتياجات المجتمعات وتحقيق رغبات المهنيين الصحيين على حد سواء.

إن ما يقرب من نصف بلدان إقليم شرق المتوسط قد اعتمدت بالفعل نماذج لممارسة طب الأسرة، وتمر هذه النماذج حالياً بمراحل مختلفة من التنفيذ. ولا يزال العديد من البلدان يتعين عليه أن يضع نماذج صالحة للتطبيق في مجال ممارسة طب

الأسرة بسبب تحدياتٍ مثل الافتقار إلى أطباء الأسرة المُدرَّبين، وانعدام التكامل بين الوقاية ورعاية الأمراض غير السارية والصحة النفسية، وضعف نُظُم المعلومات والترصد.

أما إطار العمل المُوصى به للنهوض بممارسة طب الأسرة من أجل تحقيق التغطية الصحية الشاملة فيتألف من خمسة مجالات رئيسية تتضمن إجراءات مُوجَّهة إلى البلدان وأخرى إلى منظمة الصحة العالمية.

1. **الحوكَمة**: تتعين إعادة توجيه النظم الصحية، وتطوير قدراتها لدعم ممارسة طب الأسرة. وعلى الحكومات أن تضمن حشد الالتزام السياسي اللازم، ووضع السياسات والتشريعات الملائمة، ونظم السداد المُسبق من أجل تقديم حزمة من الخدمات الصحية الأساسية من خلال نهج طب الأسرة.

2. **التوسع في برامج التدريب على طب الأسرة**: يتعين إرساء تخصص طب الأسرة وتعزيزه بهدف زيادة أعداد أطباء الأسرة المُجازين. وكترتيب انتقالي، توجد حاجة إلى برامج تأهيلية مناسبة لتحويل الممارسين العامِّين إلى أطباء أسرة.

3. **التمويل**: لا بد أن تقوم البلدان بتعزيز التمويل، وتقدير تكاليف حزم الخدمات الصحية الأساسية، ومباشرة الشراء الاستراتيجي.

4. **تكامل الخدمات وضمان جودتها**: ينبغي تقديم مجموعة من الخدمات الصحية المُنتقاة بعناية والمضمونة الجودة بطريقة متكاملة من خلال ممارسة طب الأسرة، على أن يدعم ذلك نظامُ إحالةٍ قوي. ويجب أن تحصل المرافق الصحية على الاعتماد.

5. **تمكين المجتمعات المحلية**: يمكن للقيادات المجتمعية والمتطوعين أن يكونوا بمنزلة جسر يربط بين الأسر ومرافق الرعاية الصحية. ويجب تعزيز المشاركة المجتمعية في الرعاية الصحية من خلال تطوير وتحسين نظم المشاركة المحلية واحترام الثقافات والمعتقدات المحلية.

المراجع

1. Boelen C. In: *Improving Health Systems: the Contribution of Family Medicine: A Guidebook*. Singapore: World Organization of Family Doctors, 2002.

2. Kidd M (ed). **Organization of Family Doctors**, *The Contribution of Family Medicine to Improving Health Systems: A Guidebook from the World* 2nd edition. London: Radcliffe Health, 2013.

3. World Health Organization. *Quality assessment of service provision at primary health care level*. World Health Organization, 2014 (unpublished).

التغطية الصحية الشاملة: تحديات وفرص تعليم العاملين في مجال الصحة

أماندا هاو

من أجل ضمان مستقبل زاهر للتغطية الصحية الشاملة، لا بد من وجود قوى عاملة صحية مُدرَّبة على تلبية شتى الاحتياجات في مراكز الرعاية الصحية الأولية، إلى جانب مهنيين صحيين ملتزمين بالعمل في مواقع الرعاية الصحية الأولية وبتلبية احتياجات جميع الناس.

وسواء أكان التدريب للأطباء أم للممرضات أم لغيرهم من العاملين الصحيين، هناك بعض المبادئ المهنية الأساسية التي تستند إليها التغطية الصحية الشاملة. أولها مبدأ الإنصاف، الذي يُعرَّف بأنه "**المبدأ والممارسة اللذان يضمنان التوزيع العادل والمُنصِف للموارد والبرامج والفرص وسلطات اتخاذ القرارات على جميع الفئات، مع مراعاة الاحتياجات والمتطلبات المختلفة**". كما أن تدريب العاملين على تقديم احتياجات الآخرين على احتياجاتهم ومعاملة الأشخاص المختلفين تماماً عنهم باحترام ورفق يتطلب مناهج تربوية مختلفة تماماً عن المناهج المتَّبعة في تدريس المهارات التقنية أو حقائق العلوم الحيوية.

وأما المبدأ الثاني فهو مبدأ **الإحاطة المعرفية العامة**[1] - فإذا كان على العاملين الصحيين أن يتصدوا لجوانب الرعاية التعزيزية والوقائية والعلاجية والتأهيلية والمُلطِّفة، فسوف يلزم أن يكتسبوا طائفة متنوعة من المعارف، وأن يكونوا على استعداد لاستخدامها، حتى داخل مجالهم أو في نطاق ممارستهم.

وأما المبدأ الثالث فهو "**التكامل**" - إذ توصي منظمة الصحة العالمية بالرعاية المتكاملة التي تُركِّز على الأشخاص،[2] ويُقصد بذلك وجود نية صادقة وقدرة على التفاعل مع الناس والمجتمعات المحلية في شتى جوانبهم الفريدة والمتنوعة، والعمل على أكبر عدد ممكن وفعَّال من الجوانب المختلفة للرعاية في وقت واحد. ويُعتبر تعلُّم التركيز على الشخص بدلاً من التركيز على المرض جانباً أساسياً من جوانب أي منهج دراسي حديث، وقد يتطلب أيضاً أساليب تعلُّم مختلفة وتقييماً مختلفاً ليصبح جزءاً متأصلاً في الممارسة المهنية.

وأما المبدأ الأخير فهو "**التحليل الأكاديمي**"، حيث يسأل العامل الصحي نفسه بانتظام عن سبب حدوث شيء ما، وينظر في قاعدة البيِّنات التي يمكن تطبيقها على المشكلة، ويبحث عن سُبلٍ لتحسين الوضع والتعلُّم من كل مشكلة تواجهه في عمله.[3]

ومن خلال العمل بهذه المبادئ الأربعة -ألا وهي الإنصاف، والإحاطة المعرفية العامة، والتكامل، والتحليل الأكاديمي- يمكننا أن ندرك لماذا يلزم أن يكون التدريب المهني الصحي الحديث مختلفاً من أجل تحقيق التغطية الصحية الشاملة.

ويؤدي القادة والمُعلِّمون المهنيون، عند حصولهم على دعم وطني ومؤسسي، دوراً حاسماً في إحداث تحوُّل في البيئة التعليمية، للتأكيد على السياق الأوسع للمشاكل الشائعة التي تحدث في جميع شرائح المجتمع، وتسليح القوى العاملة المستقبلية بما تحتاج إليه لتكون مؤهَّلة ومتحمسة لتلبية احتياجات الأشخاص والسكان في المجتمعات التي سيخدمونها. ويتطلب ذلك حدوث تغيير في المناهج الدراسية والأساليب التعليمية وثقافة التدريب - فضلاً عن تغيير جوانب أخرى في المنظومة. وبوجد في إقليم شرق المتوسط كثير من الأطباء السريريين والمُعلِّمين ذوي الخبرة، بالإضافة إلى بعض النماذج الناضجة للتغطية الصحية الشاملة.

ومن المبادئ الجوهرية التي تقوم عليها الإصلاحات: الإنصاف، ومنح الأولوية للممارسة العامة، وتطوير التركيز على الأشخاص مع تكامل الرعاية المُقدَّمة إلى الأفراد لتلبية احتياجاتهم، وتمكين الطلاب على جميع المستويات من التعلم من أشخاص ومجتمعات محلية على أرض الواقع، وضمان فهمهم لكيفية تحقيق النظم الصحية للتغطية الصحية الشاملة.

وقد يلزم تحديد الأعداد المُستهدَفة من المطلوب التحاقهم بكليات الطب والتمريض، لا سيما الذين سيعملون في الرعاية الأولية

والخطوط الأمامية بمواقع تلقِّي الرعاية الخارجية، فضلاً عن المساءلة عن تحقيق هذه الأهداف، لكي تتوفر لكل نظام صحي القوى العاملة المناسبة في المكان المناسب بالمهارات والسلوكيات المناسبة. ومن المهم النظر في معايير الاختيار وتوقعات المُنضمين إلى القوى العاملة الصحية.

ومن الضروري أيضاً إعداد المناهج الدراسية اللازمة لبناء المهارات المهنية ومهارات التواصل فضلاً عن المناهج الدراسية الخاصة بالعلوم الحيوية والأمراض. وتجب زيادة التواصل المباشر مع المريض، وزيادة الاستفادة من مواقع التعلُّم الموجودة خارج المستشفيات الكبرى.

ولا بد من اتخاذ إجراءات على مستويات متعددة، وإيجاد زخم، حتى لو كانت القدرات محدودة في البداية. وهذه الإجراءات تشمل الدعوة والمناصرة، وتنمية مهارات القوى العاملة الحالية، والتحفيز على الابتكار ومكافأة المبتكرين، والتعاون مع الطلاب وأعضاء هيئة التدريس والمهنيين الصحيين والمرضى على تنفيذ التغييرات اللازمة.

ويجب التصدي في الوقت نفسه للمخاطر، ومنها هجرة المهنيين الصحيين المُدرَّبين من البلدان ذات الدخل المنخفض والمتوسط إلى البلدان ذات الدخل المرتفع، ويجب على العاملين في جميع التخصصات الطبية أن يحترم ويدعم بعضهم بعضاً في مجالَي الرعاية الأولية والثانوية على حد سواء.

ويجب تشجيع الجهات المسؤولة (وهي في الغالب الجامعات، ووزارة الصحة أو وزارة التعليم أو كلتاهما، والجمعيات المهنية، وهيئات الاعتماد) على مواءمة برامجهم مع الهدف الاستراتيجي العام المتمثل في تحقيق التغطية الصحية الشاملة.

المراجع

1. Howe A, for the Royal College of General Practitioners. *Why expertise in whole person medicine matters*. London; RCGP: 2012. http://www.rcgp.org.uk/policy/rcgp-policy-areas/~/media/Files/Policy/A-Z-policy/Medical-Generalism-Why_expertise_in_whole_person_medicine_matters.ashx (جرى الاطلاع عليه في 18/1/3).

2. إطار الخدمات الصحية المتكاملة التي تركز على الناس. جمعية الصحة العالمية، 2016. http://apps.who.int/gb/ebwha/pdf_files/WHA69/A69_39-en.pdf?ua=1 (جرى الاطلاع عليه في 18/1/14).

3. Greenhalgh T, Douglas HR. Experiences of general practitioners and practice nurses of training courses in evidence-based health care: a qualitative study. *British Journal of General Practice*. 1999; 49: 536-540.

الرعاية الأولية الاستباقية: دمج الصحة العامة والرعاية الأولية
سلمان رواف، إليزابيث دوبوا، ميس رحيم، ديفيد رواف

ركّز إعلان أستانا لعام 2018 من جديد على ما أُعلن عنه في ألما آتا قبل 40 سنة، ألا وهو الدور الحاسم للرعاية الأولية في بلوغ هدف منظمة الصحة العالمية المتعلق بتحقيق الصحة للجميع، ومعالجة أوجه عدم المساواة، وتحقيق التغطية الصحية الشاملة.[1،2]

وإن كانت الرعاية الأولية تؤدي إلى تعزيز الحصول على الخدمات الصحية، وتحقيق نتائج صحية أفضل، وانخفاض عدد المرضى في المستشفيات وعدد زيارات أقسام الطوارئ، فإنها يمكن أيضاً أن تساعد على التصدي للأثر السلبي الذي قد تتركه الظروف الاقتصادية السيئة على الصحة.[3،4] ولكن الرعاية الأولية التقليدية، كما نعرفها، تركز على خدمات الرعاية الصحية الشخصية واستمرارية الرعاية. كما أن "النموذج المرضي" العلاجي لسبعينيات القرن العشرين، الذي لا يزال يُمارَس في بلدان كثيرة، يشهد في الوقت الحالي تغييراً سريعاً. والتغيرات السكانية والوبائية –مثل التقدّم في السن، والنمو السكاني، وتزايد عبء الأمراض المزمنة وغير السارية، وتعدد الأمراض– إلى جانب أوجه التقدم التكنولوجي تُوجّهان دفّة تحوّل الرعاية الأولية بعيداً عن النموذج الطبي القديم. وتقتضي هذه النقلة النوعية أن تُركّز الرعاية الأولية على الوقاية ونوعية المعيشة، وأن تحثّ على اتباع نهج استباقي لإدارة السكان يستهدف الأفراد والجماعات الأكثر تأثراً بالمُحدِّدات الهيكلية للصحة. ويتطلب تحقيقُ الفعالية وجودَ روابط قوية بين الصحة العامة والرعاية الأولية.

ولا يوجد نظام صحي يتسم بالكمال، فلكل نموذج مواطن قوته وضعفه. ولكننا نعلم أيضاً أن النُظُم الأكثر فاعلية هي تلك النُظُم القادرة على حماية صحة السكان ككل.[5] ومن المستحيل بلوغ ذلك دون تحقيق التغطية الصحية الشاملة من خلال رعاية أولية شاملة وفعالة لا تركز على المرض فحسب، بل تركز أيضاً على الصحة وكيفية تحسينها. ولذلك، لا بد أن تكون للصحة العامة وظيفةٌ استباقية قوية في إطار الرعاية الأولية من أجل حماية الصحة وتعزيزها على المستويين الجماعي والفردي والوقاية من الأمراض.[6]

ويمكن دمج الصحة العامة في الرعاية الأولية بوسائل متنوعة، منها: نقل المهنيين العاملين في مجال الصحة العامة إلى مواقع الرعاية الأولية، وإنشاء حزم شاملة واستباقية تتضمن مجموعة كبيرة من تدخلات الصحة العامة على المستويين السكاني والفردي، وتقديم الرعاية الأولية داخل مواقع الصحة العامة، ودمج حوافز الصحة العامة في الرعاية الأولية، والشروع في تقديم تدريب في مجال الصحة العامة لموظفي الرعاية الأولية وأطبائها وممرضيها.[7]

إن الصحة العامة والرعاية الأولية متلازمتان بطبيعتهما، وينبغي أن يتكاملا على المستوى الأكاديمي ومستوى تقديم الخدمات على حد سواء. والرعاية الأولية الاستباقية والشاملة والمتكاملة تنقذ الأرواح، وتقلل من عبء المرض، وتحسن نوعية المعيشة. كما أنها وسيلة مهمة لتحسين الإنتاجية، وتعزيز جودة الخدمات، وتوفير خدمة سلِسة، وتحقيق تغطية صحية شاملة.[8] وفي ظل هذه الأدلة الدامغة، فإن تغيير السياسات وتنفيذها يجب أن يكونا على وجه السرعة.

المراجع

1. World Health Organization and United Children's Fund. Declaration of Astana. Geneva: WHO, 2018. https://www.who.int/docs/default-source/primary-health/declaration/gcphc-declaration.pdf (جرى الاطلاع عليه في 20 كانون الأول/ديسمبر 2019)

2. الرعاية الصحية الأولية: الآن أكثر من أي وقت مضى. التقرير الخاص بالصحة في العالم 2008. جنيف: منظمة الصحة العالمية: 2008 https://www.who.int/whr/2008/ar/. (جرى الاطلاع عليه في 10 تشرين الأول 2018).

3. Kane RL, Keckhafer G, Flood S, Bershadsky B, Siadaty MS. The effect of Evercare on hospital use. J Am Geriatr. 2003;51:1427–34. doi: 10.1046/j.1532-5415.2003.51461

4. Shi L. The impact of primary care: a focused review. Scientifica (Cairo). 2012;2012:43289. Doi: 10.6064/2012/432892

5. Wanless D. Securing good health for the whole population. Final report. London: HMSO; 2004 https://www.southampton.gov.uk/moderngov/documents/s19272/prevention-appx%201%20wanless%20summary.pdf (جرى الاطلاع عليه في 20 كانون الثاني/يناير 2019)

6. Rawaf S. A proactive general practice: integrating public health into primary care. London J Prim Care (Abingdon). 2018; 10:17–8. doi: 10.1080/17571472.2018.1445946

7. Rawaf S. Medico de familia na saude publica (Family physicians and public health). In: Gusso G, Lopes JMC, editors. Tratado de medicina de familia e communidade: principios, formaco et practica (Treatise on family and community medicine: principles, training and practice). Porto Alegre: Artmed Editora Ltda; 2012. Volume 1:19–27.

8. Baker R, Honeyford K, Levene LS, Mainous AG, Jones DR, Bankart MJ, et al. Population characteristics, mechanisms of primary care and premature mortality in England: a cross-sectional study. BMJ Open. 2016;6:e009981. doi:10.1136/ bmjopen-2015-009981

المعلومات الصحية في مجالَي الرعاية الأولية وممارسة طب الأسرة: المفهوم، والوضع، ورؤية لإقليم شرق المتوسط

آرش رشيديان، هنري فيكتور دكتور، إيمان عبد الكريم حسن علي، عزة محمد بدر

يُعدّ نظام المعلومات الصحية "جهداً متكاملاً لجمع المعلومات الصحية ومعالجتها والإبلاغ عنها والاسترشاد بها في وضع السياسات وعمل البرامج والبحوث".[1] ويُعتبر نظام المعلومات الصحية إحدى اللبنات الأساسية التي يتكون منها أي نظام صحي. فهو يُمكِّن متخذي القرارات على جميع مستويات النظام الصحي من الوقوف على التحديات الصحية وتوزيع الموارد الشحيحة على النحو الأمثل لتحقيق تحسينات صحية. كما أن نظام المعلومات الصحية القوي الذي يُقدِّم في الوقت المناسب بيانات موثوقة ذات جودة عالية أحد العوامل العديدة التي تُمكِّن راسمي السياسات من اتخاذ قرارات مُسندة بالبيّنات.

وتأتي البيانات والمعلومات الصحية من منبعين رئيسيين، ألا وهما: مصادر البيانات السكانية (التعدادات، تسجيل الأحوال المدنية، المسوح الأسرية)، ومصادر البيانات المؤسسية (مسوح المرافق، سجلات المرافق، سجلات الأفراد).[2] وتُعتبر بيانات نظم المعلومات الصحية الروتينية، التي تُعرف أيضاً باسم نظم معلومات المرافق الصحية والمجتمعات المحلية، العماد الذي يقوم عليه التخطيط الجزئي على مستوى المرافق، واتخاذ القرارات وتخصيص الموارد وإعداد الاستراتيجية الصحية على مستوى أعلى (مثل مستوى المناطق والأقاليم والمستوى الوطني). ويتألف نظام المعلومات الصحية الروتيني من البيانات التي تُجمع على فترات منتظمة في المرافق والمؤسسات الصحية العامة والخاصة والمجتمعية. وتتيح هذه البيانات فرصة لدراسة التغيرات التي تحدث في الوضع الصحي، والخدمات الصحية، والموارد الصحية.

ورغم الاهتمام المتجدد ببيانات نظم المعلومات الصحية الروتينية والاستثمارات الكبرى فيها من أجل وضع برامج تقودها البلدان ورسم السياسات، فهناك عقبات رئيسية تحول دون استخدام هذه البيانات على نحو جيد وفعال. وتتعلق إحدى المشاكل المشتركة في كثير من المواقع بتأخُّر تقديم التقارير، بما في ذلك عدم اكتمال أو عدم دقة البيانات المُقدَّمة من المناطق والمرافق الصحية. فهذه المشاكل التي تتعلق بجودة البيانات تُقوّض المصداقية وتؤثر سلباً على استخدام المؤشرات المستندة إلى نظم المعلومات الصحية الروتينية. ولكن توجد أساليب فعالة وجديدة ومبتكرة لتحسين بيانات نظم المعلومات الصحية الروتينية، خاصةً في البلدان ذات الدخل المنخفض وذات الدخل المتوسط، وتكون هذه الأساليب في الغالب باستخدام تكنولوجيا المعلومات. وقد أسفرت هذه الأساليب عن تحسينات كبيرة في جودة البيانات من خلال الاستفادة من نظم البيانات الإلكترونية المتاحة لتعزيز جمع البيانات ومعالجتها وتحليلها واستخدام المعلومات.[4] كما أدت تقييمات جودة البيانات وخطط التحسين الناشئة عنها إلى التوسع في الاسترشاد ببيانات نظم المعلومات الصحية الروتينية عند اتخاذ القرارات.

وقد أتاح تطبيق نظم المعلومات القائمة على المرافق فرصاً لجمع المعلومات المتعلقة بفعالية التدخلات، وإدارة العلاج، والمخرجات ذات الصلة. فعند جمع هذه البيانات، يمكن استخدامها لأغراض كثيرة متنوعة، منها إدارة رعاية المرضى، الترصد الوبائي، رصد البرامج الخاصة بتدخلات محددة، تقييمات الجودة. وعلاوة على ذلك، قد تكون هذه البيانات مفيدة في استكمال مصادر بيانات أخرى لاكتشاف الفاشيات والإبلاغ عنها.

ورغم أنه لا غنى عن نظم المعلومات الصحية من أجل التنفيذ الفعال لنهوج الرعاية الأولية وممارسة طب الأسرة، فإن بلدان إقليم شرق المتوسط تختلف اختلافاً كبيراً في أساليب جمع المعلومات واستخدامها ومراقبة نظم المعلومات. وحتى في البلدان التي تتشابه نماذجها الأولية الخاصة بالرعاية الصحية الأولية، بناءً على توصيات منظمة الصحة العالمية، تختلف نظم المعلومات الصحية إلى حد بعيد. وقد يرجع ذلك، جزئياً، إلى أنه لم يُقدَّم، من البداية، أسلوبٌ منهجي لتطبيق نظم المعلومات الصحية إلى جانب الرعاية الأولية، ولم تُحدَّد بالتفصيل الخصائص الدنيا لنظام المعلومات الصحية الفعال.

وعلى الرغم من هذه الاختلافات، فإن نظم المعلومات الصحية في نظم الرعاية الأولية لشتى البلدان توفر رؤية كافية للعمل

وبعض الفرص للتعلم. ولدى منظمة الصحة العالمية خطةُ عملٍ لتحسين نظم المعلومات الصحية في إقليم شرق المتوسط. وتشتمل خطة العمل هذه على إطار إقليمي لجمع المؤشرات الأساسية والإبلاغ عنها، وخطة لتحسين النظم الوطنية للتسجيل المدني والإحصاءات الحيوية، مع التركيز على تسجيل الوفيات والإشهاد الدقيق على أسباب الوفاة، ونموذج لإجراء تقييمات شاملة لنظام المعلومات الصحية.[5-6]ويولي النموذج الأخير اهتماماً كافياً بتنظيم نظم المعلومات الصحية الوطنية، بما في ذلك تنظيمها في مجال الرعاية الأولية، والأمل معقود على أن يساعد ذلك على توحيد الإجراءات لدعم التحسين المستمر لنظم الرعاية الأولية.

المراجع

1. Lippeveld T. Routine health information systems: The glue of a unified health system. [Keynote address] Workshop on Issues and Innovation in Routine Health Information in Developing Countries. Potomac, Washington, DC, 14–16 March 2001.

2. *Health Metrics Network.* Assessing the National Health Information System: An Assessment Tool Version 4.00. *Geneva: World Health Organization, 2008.*

3. Mutale W, Chintu N, Amoroso C, Awoonor-Williams K, Phillips J, Baynes C, et al. Improving health information systems for decision making across five sub-Saharan African countries: Implementation strategies from the African Health Initiative. *BMC Health Services Research, 2013; 13(Suppl 2): S9.* متاح على: http://www.biomedcentral.com/1472–6963/13/S2/S9 [جرى الاطلاع عليه في 17 شباط/فبراير 2018].

4. Wagenaar BH, Sherr K, Fernandes Q, Wagenaar AC. Using routine health information systems for well-designed health evaluations in low-and middle-income countries. *Health Policy and Planning, 2016; 31(1): 129–135.*

5. Alwan A, Ali M, Aly E, Badr A, Doctor H, Mandil A, Rashidian A, Shideed O. Strengthening national health information systems: Challenges and response. *Eastern Mediterranean Health Journal, 2016; 22(11): 840–850.*

6. **منظمة الصحة العالمية. الاستراتيجية الإقليمية لتحسين نظم تسجيل الأحوال المدنية والإحصاءات الحيوية 2014-2019. القاهرة: المكتب الإقليمي لمنظمة الصحة العالمية لشرق المتوسط. 2014.**

إدماج الأمراض غير السارية في الرعاية الصحية الأولية بإقليم شرق المتوسط

سليم سلامة، جيما ليونز، هبة فؤاد، شانون باركلي، أزموس همريتش

تمثل الأمراض غير السارية عبئاً ثقيلاً في إقليم شرق المتوسط، إذ تتسبب في 63% من جميع الوفيات المسجلة. ومن المتوقع أن تصل هذه النسبة إلى ما يقرب من 70% بحلول عام 2030. ويتطلب النهوض بالعبء الاجتماعي والاقتصادي الذي تفرضه هذه الظروف نهجاً يشمل الحكومة بأكملها والمجتمع بأسره، من أجل إعداد استجابات وطنية قُطرية تتضمن تدابير وقائية شاملة لجميع السكان، مصحوبة بخدمات صحية قادرة على الكشف المبكر عن الأمراض غير السارية وعوامل الخطر المرتبطة بها والتدبير العلاجي لهذه الأمراض، وذلك من خلال إيلاء الأولوية لأكثر التدخلات فعالية من حيث التكلفة وإدماج هذه التدخلات، المعروفة باسم "أفضل الصفقات" التي توصي بها منظمة الصحة العالمية.

ويشدد إطار منظمة الصحة العالمية لعام 2016 بشأن "الخدمات الصحية المتكاملة التي تُركِّز على الناس" على أهمية تمحور الرعاية الصحية الأولية حول الاحتياجات الشاملة للناس، بدلاً من اقتصارها على أمراض محددة. وعلاوة على ذلك، فإن الزخم الذي أحدثته أهداف التنمية المستدامة، والجهود التي تُبذَل حالياً لتوسيع نطاق التغطية الصحية الشاملة، يُسلِّطان الضوء من جديد على التدخلات الأساسية الخاصة بالأمراض غير السارية التي يجب إدماجها في حزم الخدمات التي تُقدَّم في بلد ما، والمستويات التي من المتوقع تقديم تلك التدخلات عليها، ومتطلبات النظم الصحية اللازمة لتقديمها، وكذلك آليات تمويل الرعاية الصحية اللازمة لضمان الحماية المالية والحد من النفقات التي يدفعها المواطنون من أموالهم.

ولا يوجد حتى الآن تعريف موحد لإدماج الأمراض غير السارية ضمن الرعاية الصحية الأولية. ولكن يمكن وصف هذا الإدماج بأنه عملية تضمين الأمراض غير السارية في الرعاية الصحية الأولية بجميع مجالات النظام الصحي. وقد حددت منظمة الصحة العالمية اللَّبِنات الأساسية التي يتكون منها النظام الصحي على النحو التالي:[1] القيادة والحوكمة، التمويل الصحي، القوى العاملة الصحية، المنتجات الطبية، اللقاحات والتكنولوجيات، المعلومات الصحية، تقديم الخدمات الصحية.

على سبيل المثال، سيشمل الإدماج على مستوى الحوكمة استراتيجيات مثل خطة وطنية تمويلية وتنفيذية لمكافحة الأمراض غير السارية تنطوي على إطار للرصد والتقييم. وأما على مستوى الموارد البشرية، فيتطلب الإدماج استراتيجيات مثل إدراج المعلومات والمهارات الخاصة بالأمراض غير السارية في عمليات تدريب القوى العاملة في مجال الرعاية الصحية الأولية وتوظيفها واستبقائها، والتركيز على العمل الجماعي المتعدد التخصصات، وتوزيع الأدوار لضمان الاستخدام المناسب للموارد المتاحة بناءً على احتياجات السكان الصحية. ومن الجدير بالذكر أن بعض المهارات والمناهج قد تكون مشتركة بين جميع الأمراض غير السارية الرئيسية الأربعة، مثل استهداف عوامل الخطر المشتركة بينها.

ورغم أن التحديات تختلف حسب مستوى الموارد ومدى تطور النظم الصحية، فقد حُدِّد عدد من التحديات المشتركة التي تعترض إدماج الأمراض غير السارية، منها: نقص التمويل، الافتقار إلى المعايير/ المبادئ التوجيهية/ البروتوكولات، عدم وجود عدد كافٍ من الموظفين وعدم تلقيهم لتدريب مناسب، انخفاض مستوى الوعي العام، عدم كفاية الأدوية والتكنولوجيات الأساسية الخاصة بالأمراض غير السارية، الميل إلى التركيز على الرعاية العلاجية، قلة الخبرة في إدماج تدخلات الاكتشاف المبكر، فضلاً عن عجز نظم المعلومات عن تقديم معلومات بشأن جودة الرعاية وأداء البرامج.

وترصد منظمة الصحة العالمية بصورة دورية قدرة الدول الأعضاء على التصدي لأوبئة الأمراض غير السارية، وذلك من خلال مسح عالمي يُعرف باسم «مسح القدرات القُطرية بشأن الأمراض غير السارية».[2] وهذا المسح العالمي الذي يُجرى منذ عام 2000 يشمل: البنية التحتية للنظام الصحي، التمويل، السياسات والخطط والاستراتيجيات، الترصد، الشراكات والتعاون المتعدد الأطراف. ويحتوي المسح على مجموعة مُحدَّدة من الأسئلة التي تُقيِّم القدرة الوطنية على علاج الأمراض غير السارية على مستوى الرعاية الصحية الأولية. ويوفر ذلك مجموعة مفيدة من المعلومات لعقد مقارنة بين أقاليم منظمة الصحة العالمية بشأن إدماج الأمراض غير السارية في الرعاية الصحية الأولية.

ويمثل تقديم خدمات الرعاية الصحية الأولية المُوجَّهة نحو الأمراض غير السارية عائقاً مشتركاً بين جميع الدول الأعضاء في إقليم شرق المتوسط، رغم وجود اختلافات في أداء النظام الصحي ومستوى الإنفاق الصحي من دولة لأخرى. وقد دأبت نظم الرعاية الصحية الأولية في الإقليم على التركيز على الأمراض السارية، والحالات الحادة الأخرى، وصحة الأمهات والأطفال. ومن ثمّ كانت الرعاية الصحية الأولية مُرتَّبة عمودياً ومُنظَّمة وفقاً لخدمات مُحدَّدة. ولم يكن هذا النظام متوافقاً مع الحاجة إلى إيلاء اعتبار شامل لزائر الرعاية الصحية الأولية، وأحواله الصحية، وأسلوب حياته طوال المراحل العمرية. ولذلك بدأت عملية تحوُّل، مما سمح للرعاية الصحية الأولية بالابتعاد عما كان يُتَّبع في الماضي من أساليب عمودية خاصة بأمراض بعينها، والاتجاه نحو رعاية أوسع تتمحور حول الناس.

وسوف يلزم توسيع نطاق أساليب الإدماج في جميع أنحاء الإقليم لكي تحقق البلدان غايات الأمم المتحدة الخاصة بالأمراض غير السارية بحلول عام 2025. ويتيح أسلوب النظام الصحي المُوضَّح طريقة منهجية للوقوف على عقبات النظام الصحي التي تحول دون الإدماج الفعال، وللتصدي تدريجياً لهذه العقبات.

المراجع

1. WHO Western Pacific Region. Health Services Development. The WHO Health Systems Framework. http://www.wpro.who.int/health_services/health_systems_framework/en/ [جرى الاطلاع عليه في 7 كانون الأول/ديسمبر 2017].

2. WHO. Noncommunicable disease and their risk factors: Assessing national capacity for the prevention and control of NCDs. http://www.who.int/ncds/surveillance/ncd-capacity/en/ [جرى الاطلاع عليه في 15 كانون الأول/ديسمبر 2017].

القوى العاملة في مجال ممارسة طب الأسرة: فرق متعددة التخصصات

فتحية جولين جيديك، أروى عويس، ميريت خليل

في إطار الجهود الرامية إلى المضي قُدُماً صوب تحقيق التغطية الصحية الشاملة، يوجد اتجاه عالمي وإقليمي نحو توفير الرعاية الأولية القائمة على ممارسة طب الأسرة. ولكن في إقليم شرق المتوسط بلدان كثيرة لا تواجه نقصاً عاماً في العاملين الصحيين فحسب، بل تواجه أيضاً تحديات في استقطاب المهنيين الصحيين وتوظيفهم واستبقائهم للعمل في مواقع الرعاية الصحية الأولية. ويؤثر ذلك تأثيراً كبيراً على توفر الخدمات التي تُقدَّم في مواقع الرعاية الأولية وسهولة الوصول إلى هذه الخدمات وجودتها، لا سيما في المناطق الريفية والنائية.

وتشدد نماذج ممارسة طب الأسرة على أهمية الفريق المتعدد التخصصات بوصفه وسيلة لتقديم رعاية أولية عالية الجودة.[1] وقد يختلف تشكيل الفريق من بلد إلى آخر حسب حزمة الخدمات الأساسية، والهياكل، والموارد، ومدى توفر الموارد البشرية.[2]

وينبغي أن ينطوي التعليم المهني الصحي على قدرٍ كافٍ من الاحتكاك بمرافق الرعاية الأولية والتدريب المجتمعي، مع تعزيز مهارات التواصل وتوكيد الذات والتفكير النقدي واتخاذ القرارات لتلبية احتياجات المجتمعات المحلية في توفير الرعاية التي تركز على المريض وإظهار مهارات الإدارة العملية والمشتركة بين المهن.[3]

ويعاني كثير من بلدان إقليم شرق المتوسط نقصاً في القوى العاملة، وانخفاضاً في مستوى الإنتاج عن الحد الأمثل، وعدم توازن في التوزيع الجغرافي والجنساني والمهاري، فضلاً عن مخاوف تتعلق بالجودة والملاءمة والأداء. ويكون هذا النقص أشد ما يكون على مستوى الرعاية الأولية. فالبلدان التي تعاني نقصاً حاداً في العاملين الصحيين قد تواجه صعوبة في نشر أعداد كافية من الأطباء والممرضات في مرافق الرعاية الأولية، خاصةً في المناطق الريفية. وفي بعض الحالات، تخلو مرافق الرعاية الأولية من أي أطباء على الإطلاق. ففي العراق على سبيل المثال، يفتقر 40% من مراكز الرعاية الصحية الأولية إلى الأطباء، ويقيم 84% من الأطباء في مناطق حضرية، ويعمل 74% من الأطباء في مستشفيات، ولا يعمل في مراكز الرعاية الصحية الأولية سوى 23%.[4، 5] وفي الصومال، لا يعمل في المواقع الريفية سوى 9% من الأطباء.[6]

ورغم استمرار زيادة التوسع الحضري على الصعيد العالمي وفي إقليم شرق المتوسط، يعيش في مناطق ريفية 60% أو أكثر من سكان بلدان الإقليم ذات الدخل المنخفض وذات الدخل المتوسط. وسوف يتطلب ضمان توفير الرعاية الأولية المناسبة القائمة على ممارسة طب الأسرة تقديم التدخلات والحوافز الضرورية لجذب المهنيين الصحيين للعمل على مستوى الرعاية الأولية. ولا يخفى على أحد أن تقديم توليفة من التدخلات التعليمية والتنظيمية والحوافز المالية، فضلاً عن الدعم المهني والشخصي، قد يساعد على تحسين نشر الموظفين واستبقائهم في مجال الرعاية الأولية وكذلك في المناطق الريفية والنائية، مما يؤدي إلى تحسين توزيع العاملين الصحيين.[7]

وتشير هذه الاتجاهات إلى أن النقص سيستمر، وأن مَيل المهنيين الصحيين إلى التخصص والعمل في المستشفيات قد يكون عقبة في طريق تعزيز الرعاية الأولية والتحوُّل إلى نماذج ممارسة طب الأسرة وتحقيق التغطية الصحية الشاملة. وتوجد حاجة ماسة إلى تدخلات تجعل الأطباء يتخصصون في طب الأسرة وتحفِّزهم على العمل على مستوى الرعاية الأولية.

وتتجاوز الرعاية الأولية القائمة على ممارسة طب الأسرة تدريب أطباء الأسرة وإدخالهم في النظام. وغالباً ما يتحول الاهتمام الشديد والجهد الكبير إلى تدريب أطباء الأسرة وزيادة عددهم، دون إيلاء اهتمام كافٍ لتدريب أعضاء الفريق الآخرين، لا سيما القوى العاملة في التمريض والقبالة.

وتُعد الحوافز المالية، وآليات الدفع الرامية إلى تحسين الأداء، والنهوض ببيئة العمل، والحصول على الأدوية والإمدادات المناسبة بعض الأمثلة المهمة للتغييرات المتعلقة بالنظام اللازمة لضمان عدم خروج القوى العاملة المدربة في مجال الرعاية الصحية الأولية خارج البلد أو عدم انتقالها إلى القطاع الخاص. وينبغي أن يكون لتغييرات النظام تأثير على سلوك كلٍّ من مُقدِّم الخدمة والمستخدم مع تحسين جودة الخدمات.

ولا يزال نموذج الرعاية الأولية القائمة على ممارسة طب الأسرة في إقليم شرق المتوسط مُفتَّتاً، ويعاني نقصاً كبيراً في الموظفين، وغير مُستغَل بالقدر الكافي. ولا بد من بذل جهود سياسية جادة، وتقديم استثمارات مالية، وتحسين التعليم المهني الصحي لتعزيز الرعاية الأولية القائمة على ممارسة طب الأسرة من أجل تكوين فريق دائم متعدد التخصصات وقادر على تلبية احتياجات السكان.

المراجع

1. Rodriguez HP, Rogers WH, Marshall RE, Safran DG. Multidisciplinary primary care teams: Effects on the quality of the clinician-patient interactions and organizational features of care. *Med Care, 2007; 45(1): 19–27*.

2. Schuetz B, Mann E, Everett W. Educating health professionals collaboratively for team-based primary care. *Health Aff (Millwood), 2010; 29(8): 1476–80*.

3. Babiker A, El Husseini M, Al Nemri A, Al Frayh A, Al Juryyan N, Faki M, et al. Health care professional development: Working as a team to improve patient care. *Sudanese J Paediatrics. 2014; 14(2): 9–16*.

4. Al Hilfi TK, Lafta R, Burnham G. Health services in Iraq. *Lancet, 2013; 381(9870): 939–48*.

5. Shukor AR, Klazinga NS, Kringos DS. Primary care in an unstable security, humanitarian, economic and political context: The Kurdistan Region of Iraq. *BMC Health Serv Res, 2017; 17(1): 592*.

6. WHO. Strategic review of the Somali health sector: Challenges and prioritized actions. متاح على: http://moh.gov.so/en/images/publication/review_somali_Health_sector.pdf [جرى الاطلاع عليه في 26 كانون الأول/ديسمبر 2017].

7. WHO. Increasing access to health workers in remote and rural areas through improved retention. متاح على: http://www.who.int/hrh/retention/guidelines/en/ [جرى الاطلاع عليه في 18 كانون الثاني 2018].

الوضع الحالي للتعليم والتدريب في مجال طب الأسرة بإقليم شرق المتوسط
واريس قدواي، جوهر واجد

يشهد طب الأسرة في الوقت الحالي توسُّعاً وانتشاراً بمعدلات متفاوتة في إقليم شرق المتوسط. ولكن عدم وجود موارد بشرية مُدرَّبة يقف حجر عثرة أمام إحراز تقدم في هذا الصدد، ويرجع ذلك في المقام الأول إلى نقص البرامج التدريبية، وعدم وجود دعم من بعض راسمي السياسات لهذا التخصص.[1] وتوجد أمثلة كثيرة لبلدان استفادت من نموذج ممارسة طب الأسرة.[2] فقد أوصيَ بتدريب 20% من جميع الأطباء في الدول الست الأعضاء في مجلس التعاون الخليجي ليتخصصوا في طب الأسرة على مدار السنوات العشر القادمة، ولكن تحقيق ذلك الهدف سيستغرق، في حالة البحرين على سبيل المثال، أكثر من 20 سنة.[3]

ولا بد أن يكون التعليم والتدريب في مجال طب الأسرة على مستوى التعليم الطبي الجامعي، والتدريب التخصصي بعد التخرج، والتدريب الذي يرمي إلى بناء قدرات القوى العاملة الطبية الحالية.

أقسام طب الأسرة والتعليم الطبي الجامعي

لا غنى عن برامج طب الأسرة في المرحلة الجامعية لتكون بمنزلة أساس لهذا التخصص. فلا بد أن يتعرف طلاب كليات الطب على هذا التخصص وأن ينظروا إليه على أنه خيار مهني جدير بالاهتمام. ولتحقيق هذا الهدف الجوهري، يجب أن توجد أقسام طب الأسرة في جميع كليات الطب. وتشير الدراسات إلى أنه في حالة بلدان مثل البحرين والمملكة العربية السعودية، يتلقى عدد كبير من خريجي كليات الطب تدريباً تخصصياً بعد التخرج في طب الأسرة، ويرجع ذلك إلى وجود أقسام طب الأسرة في كلياتهم وتدريس طب الأسرة في المرحلة الجامعية. كما أن التعليم الطبي في المرحلة الجامعية بمعظم المؤسسات التعليمية في إقليم شرق المتوسط يرتكز إلى حد بعيد على المستشفيات، في حين أنه ينبغي أن يتضمن بقدر كبير من الأنشطة المجتمعية.[1]

التدريب التخصصي بعد التخرج في مجال طب الأسرة

في إقليم شرق المتوسط نقصٌ عام في البرامج التدريبية التي يمكن أن تُخرج موارد بشرية مُدرَّبة للعمل في أقسام طب الأسرة. ويمكن استخلاص استراتيجيات من النماذج الحالية التي نجحت في تقديم تدريب في مجال طب الأسرة في فترة زمنية قصيرة، ومنها مشروع برايمافيمد (Primafamed) الذي أشرك 10 جامعات من ثمانية من بلدان جنوب الصحراء الكبرى في تدريب أطباء الأسرة على مدى سنتين ونصف السنة.[4] وقد اتبع هذا المشروع نهجاً استراتيجياً يقوم على نماذج مأخوذة عن بلدان العالم المتقدم. وقد استفاد السودان من بلدان إقليم شرق المتوسط من هذا النموذج.

دورة تدريبية قصيرة لبناء قدرات الممارسين العامِّين

تزعم بلدان عديدة في إقليم شرق المتوسط أن لديها دورات دراسية قصيرة في طب الأسرة للممارسين العامِّين الحاليين، وأن مدتها تصل إلى عام. وقد ظهرت الحاجة إلى مثل هذه الدورات القصيرة في مجال طب الأسرة. وغالباً ما تُقام هذه الدورات في القطاع العام، ويبدو أنها تلبي احتياجات ملحة قصيرة المدى. ويجب إشراك القطاع الخاص أيضاً في هذا المسعى. وهناك مخاوف بشأن مدى مأمونية تحوُّل أطباء الأسرة إلى أطباء سريريين بعد اجتياز هذه الدورات القصيرة. وتحتاج القضايا المتعلقة بالمقررات الدراسية والتقييم والاعتماد إلى مزيد من التعزيز. ويمكن أن يكون اعتماد البرامج التدريبية إما على المستوى الوطني، كاعتمادها من الهيئة السعودية للتخصصات الصحية في المملكة العربية السعودية، أو على المستوى الإقليمي، كاعتمادها من المجلس العربي لطب الأسرة والمجتمع. ويجب أن تدعو منظمة الصحة العالمية إلى عقد دورات دراسية قصيرة بشأن تحسين قدرات الممارسين العامِّين لضمان جودة ممارسة الذين يجتازون هذه الدورات، وأن هذه الدورات مسموح بها لفترة زمنية محدودة إلى أن يُنشأ عددٌ كافٍ من البرامج التدريبية التخصصية بعد التخرج في مجال طب الأسرة. وتوجد أيضاً حاجة إلى دورات التعليم الطبي المستمر

للنهوض بمعايير أطباء الأسرة الممارسين في جميع أنحاء الإقليم.[5]

وتعاني معظم الدول الأعضاء في إقليم شرق المتوسط نقصاً شديداً في الموارد البشرية الصحية، خاصةً في طب الأسرة. ويجب أن تبذل الدول الأعضاء جهوداً متضافرة لتقديم التعليم والتدريب في مجال طب الأسرة على المستوى الجامعي والدراسات العليا والتطوير المهني المستمر. وستحتاج معظم البلدان في إقليم شرق المتوسط إلى إجراء تحوُّل كبير لتعزيز نُظُم الرعاية الصحية الخاصة بها وتحويلها من نُظُم مستندة إلى المستشفيات وتُركِّز على علاج الأمراض إلى نُظُم مجتمعية تُركِّز على تقديم خدمات صحية أساسية وتعزيزية ووقائية وعلاجية شاملة إلى جميع شعوبها.

المراجع

1. World Health Organization, Eastern Mediterranean Region Working Paper. Current Status of Family Medicine Education and Training in Eastern Mediterranean Region, 2014.

2. Kidd M. The Contribution of Family Medicine to Improving Health Systems. A Guidebook from the World Organization of Family Doctors (2nd edition), 2013. New York: Radcliffe Publishing London.

3. Alnasir FAL. Family medicine in the Arab world? Is it a luxury? Journal of the Bahrain Medical Society, 2009; 21(1): 191–192.

4. Flinkenflögel M, Essuman A, Patrick Chege P, Ayankogbe O, and Maeseneer JD. Family medicine training in sub-Saharan Africa: South-South cooperation in the Primafamed project as strategy for development. Family Practice, 2014; 31(4): 427–436.

5. Anwar H, Batty H. Continuing medical education strategy for primary health care physicians in Oman: lessons to be learnt. Oman Medical Journal, 2007; 22(3): 33–35.

الاستفادة من التقنية في تحوُّل الممارسين العامين إلى نموذج ممارسة طب الأسرة

غسان حمادة، منى عثمان، حسين حمام

اعتمد المكتب الإقليمي لمنظمة الصحة العالمية لشرق المتوسط مفهوم ممارسة طب الأسرة من أجل تحقيق التغطية الصحية الشاملة.[1] ونتناول في هذا الفصل استخدام أدوات التعلم الإلكتروني لتحوُّل الممارسين العامِّين ذوي الخبرة إلى نموذج الرعاية القائم على ممارسة طب الأسرة.

وتتميز ممارسة طب الأسرة بثماني سمات، ألا وهي تقديم رعاية عامة، وأولية، ومستمرة، وشاملة، ومُنسَّقة، وتعاونية، مع التوجه نحو الأسرة، والتوجه نحو المجتمع.[2] ومن المتوقع أن يؤدي وجود منهج دراسي لتدريب الممارسين العامِّين أو أطباء الأسرة إلى تيسير اكتساب المهارات والقدرات الأساسية التي حددتها المنظمة العالمية لأطباء الأسرة، ألا وهي: إدارة الرعاية الأولية، الرعاية التي تركز على الشخص، مهارات حل المشاكل، النهج الشامل، التوجه المجتمعي، النهج الكُلّي.[3]

ويتمثل التحدي الرئيسي الذي يعترض تنفيذ ممارسة طب الأسرة بإقليم شرق المتوسط في محدودية عدد البرامج المتاحة للتدريب على طب الأسرة وقلة عدد الأطباء الممارسين لطب الأسرة.[4] ورغم أن زيادة عدد البرامج التدريبية هي النهج المُفضَّل للتصدي لهذا التحدي، فإن الارتقاء بمهارات الممارسين العامِّين في نموذج ممارسة طب الأسرة من خلال برامج التطوير المهني التأهيلية يمثل خياراً بديلاً.[4] وقد اعتمدت بلدان عديدة برامج إعفائية أو تأهيلية تُفضي إلى الحصول على دبلومات أو شهادات.

وقد أحدثت التطورات التقنية ثورةً في طرق التدريس التقليدية من خلال تمكين المُعلِّمين من تنظيم فصول دراسية افتراضية لجمهور أكبر حسب الزمان والمكان المناسبين للمتعلم. ويُعدُّ هذا النمط من التعلم مثالياً للمهنيين العاملين. وأما الاقتصار على التدريب المُقدَّم عبر الإنترنت فلم يحظَ بالإقرار حتى الآن، لا سيما في القطاعات الصحية.[5] وربما يكون السبب هو أن معظم الجامعات لا تزال تستخدم "التعلم المختلط"، الذي يجمع بين التدريب عبر الإنترنت والأنشطة التي تُقام وجهاً لوجه.

وقد خاطب المكتب الإقليمي لمنظمة الصحة العالمية لشرق المتوسط قسم طب الأسرة في المركز الطبي للجامعة الأمريكية في بيروت لإعداد دورة مُحدَّثة بشأن "الممارسة العامة المتقدمة". وتستهدف هذه الدورة الممارسين العامِّين الذين لم يتلقوا أي تدريب مهني أو تخصصي قبل بدء الممارسة، وهي مكملة للخبرة التي اكتسبها هؤلاء الممارسون في حياتهم المهنية، وتسعى إلى استعادة تركيزهم على المكونات الرئيسية لنموذج ممارسة طب الأسرة.

وتستمر الدورة 24 أسبوعاً، وتُستخدم فيها منصة "موودل" (MOODLE) لإدارة التعلُّم بشكل مختلط يتلاءم مع مواعيد عمل الممارسين العامِّين ويسمح بالتفاعل المستمر عبر الإنترنت بين المُعلمين والمتدربين.

وتتضمن الدورة جلسة توجيهية، وأربع وحدات تعليمية (بما في ذلك عروض تقديمية ومناقشات عبر شبكة الإنترنت، وجلسات تدريب ميداني، ومراجعات مباشرة)، وفترة اختبار. ويعتمد تقييم المُتدربين على التقييم التكويني والتقييم الختامي. ولا بد من وجود مدير للدورة واختصاصي في تقنية المعلومات من أجل إقامة الدورة على نحو سليم.

وقد أُقيمت الدورة لأول مرة في عام 2017 بمشاركة 16 ممارساً عامّاً ممن يعملون مع وكالة الأمم المتحدة لإغاثة وتشغيل اللاجئين (الأونروا) في لبنان. وقُسِّم الممارسون العامُّون إلى ثلاث مجموعات، خُصِّص لكل مجموعة منها مُعلم. وقام المعلمون بمتابعة المتدربين أسبوعياً عبر الإنترنت، وأجروا تدريباً ميدانياً مرتين لكل وحدة تعليمية. وكان يُنتظَر من الممارسين العامِّين استكمال عروض تقديمية واختبارات قصيرة عبر الإنترنت كل أسبوع، وأداء واجب دراسي واحد في كل وحدة تعليمية، وحضور جلسة مراجعة مباشرة واحدة لكل وحدة. وفي ختام الدورة المكوَّنة من أربع وحدات، جرى تقييم الممارسين العامِّين من خلال اختبار تحريري نهائي وفحص سريري موضوعي مُنظَّم (OSCE). وأُجريت الدورة بسلاسة، وأظهرت التعقيبات المُقدَّمة من الممارسين العامِّين قدراً كبيراً من الرضا عن محتوى الدورة وطريقة التدريب.

وتُعدّ التكنولوجيا وسيلة مجدية لتحوُّل الممارسين العامّين إلى نموذج ممارسة طب الأسرة. وتُقدَّم هذه الدورة باعتبارها تطويراً مهنياً مستمراً ومُنظَّماً تقدمه إحدى الجامعات في مجال الممارسة العامة. ومن أجل تسريع التحوُّل إلى نموذج ممارسة طب الأسرة في جميع أنحاء الإقليم في المستقبل، ينبغي للهيئات المسؤولة عن منح تراخيص التخصص أن تعتمد برنامجاً تأهيلياً كاملاً إلى أن يُنشأ عددٌ كافٍ من برامج التدريب العملي المتكاملة.

المراجع

1. EMRO. Conceptual and strategic approach to family practice: Towards universal health coverage through family practice in the Eastern Mediterranean Region. 2014; متاح على: http://applications.emro.who.int/dsaf/EMROPUB_2014_EN_1783.pdf [جرى الاطلاع عليه في 17 تشرين الثاني/نوفمبر 2017].

2. Kidd, M.R. The Contribution of Family Medicine to Improving Health Systems: A guidebook from the World Organization of Family Doctors (2nd edition), 2013. London, New York: Radcliffe Pub. xxvii, 293 p.

3. WONCA. The European Definition of General Practice/Family Medicine. 2011 [جرى الاطلاع عليه في 17 تشرين الثاني/نوفمبر 2017].

4. المكتب الإقليمي لمنظمة الصحة العالمية لشرق المتوسط. توسيع نطاق ممارسة طب الأسرة: التقدُّم المُحرَز من أجل تحقيق التغطية الصحية الشاملة. اللجنة الإقليمية لشرق المتوسط 2016؛ ش م/ ل إ /63/ مناقشة تقنية.1 تنقيح 1 [جرى الاطلاع عليه في 17 تشرين الثاني/نوفمبر 2017].

5. McCutcheon, K. et al., A systematic review evaluating the impact of online or blended learning vs. face-to-face learning of clinical skills in undergraduate nurse education. *Journal of Advanced Nursing, 2015, 71(2): 255–270.*

قياس جودة الرعاية الصحية الأولية: مبادرة إقليمية في شرق المتوسط

منذر لطيف، ليزا هيرشهورن، عزيز شيخ، ثمين صديقي

من أجل تعزيز قياس الرعاية الصحية الأولية لدفع عجلة التغيير، شرع المكتب الإقليمي لمنظمة الصحة العالمية لشرق المتوسط في اتخاذ إجراءات تهدف إلى تحديد واختبار مجموعة أساسية من المؤشرات لتحسين جودة تقديم الرعاية الصحية من خلال تحسين القياس مما يُفضي إلى إدخال تحسينات. واشتملت هذه الإجراءات على سلسلة استراتيجية من الأنشطة، منها استعراض المؤلفات والدراسات السابقة، ومساهمة الخبراء، وإجراء اختبار تجريبي، وعقد مؤتمرات إقليمية لتبادل المعلومات، وتكرار مجموعة من التدابير الأساسية.

واشتملت منهجية هذه الإجراءات على سلسلة من الخطوات، منها إنشاء إطار ينطوي على استمرارية الرعاية الصحية وإطار دونابيديان التقليدي.[1] ثم أُضيفت إلى ذلك ستة أبعاد أساسية من أبعاد الجودة.[2] ثم جرى اختيار مؤشرات جودة الرعاية، مع مراعاة الخصائص الحاسمة الثلاث لأي مؤشر، ألا وهي: الأهمية، الصلاحية، الجدوى. واشتملت عملية الاختيار على اختيار المؤشر الأولي من خلال استعراض سريع لنطاق المؤلفات والدراسات الحالية، مع البحث باستخدام مصطلحات "جودة الرعاية" و"المؤشرات" و"التدابير"، وإعداد مصفوفة مؤشرات مرشحة. واستُكمل استعراض المؤلفات والدراسات بمساهمات من خبراء في مجال جودة الرعاية والرعاية الأولية من جميع أنحاء إقليم شرق المتوسط. وأعقب ذلك التواصل بطريقة دلفي الإلكترونية (eDelphi) مع 27 خبيراً من داخل الإقليم وخارجه لاستعراض المؤشرات المرشحة.[3] ثم أُجري اختبار تجريبي على نطاق ضيق في ثلاثة من مرافق الرعاية الصحية الأولية في مصر ومركزين من مراكز الرعاية الصحية الأولية التابعة لوكالة الأمم المتحدة لإغاثة وتشغيل اللاجئين الفلسطينيين (الأونروا) في الأردن. وقد أدى هذا العمل إلى تنقيح مجموعة المؤشرات ذات الأولوية، وأسفر عن تعديلات مقترحة لتعريفات تشغيلية. ومن أجل توسيع نطاق الاختبار، وُضعت قائمة نهائية تضم 34 مؤشراً[4]، وتشمل ستة من مجالات الجودة (الإتاحة، الإنصاف، السلامة، الكفاءة، الفعالية، التركيز على المريض)، مع تقسيم كل مجال إلى ثلاث فئات فرعية (الهيكل، العملية، المخرجات). وأعِدّت مجموعة أدوات لمواصلة اختبار جدوى قياس المؤشرات، وتوفُّر البيانات، والتحديات والفجوات. وجرى قياس مجموعة المؤشرات المُحدَّدة باستخدام مجموعة الأدوات من خلال عملية تتألف من خمس خطوات في عشرة مرافق بكل بلد من البلدان الأربعة (إيران، الأردن، عمان، تونس) ومن خلال مرافق تديرها الأونروا.

وأظهرت نتائج الاختبار في البلدان الأربعة ومع الأونروا وجود تفاوت كبير داخل البلدان وفيما بينها بشأن كلٍّ من توفُّر البيانات والنتائج. وفيما يخص التركيز على المريض، لم تكن توجد بيانات كافية إلا لدى بلدين اثنين، بنسبة 44% و64%، في حين أن 53% و77% في هذين البلدين كانوا على دراية بحقوق المرضى ومسؤولياتهم.

ورغم أن معدلات تحصين الأطفال الذين تقل أعمارهم عن 23 شهراً كانت مرتفعة بوجه عام (من 82% إلى 100%)، كان تطعيم الإنفلونزا أقل بكثير. وكانت النسبة المئوية لمرضى ارتفاع ضغط الدم المسجَّلين الذين لديهم ضغط الدم أكثر من 90/140 في زيارتَي المتابعة الأخيرتين تتراوح بين 32% و73%، أما مرضى السكري المُسجَّلين الذين تقل نسبة خضاب الدم السكري (Hba1c) لديهم عن 7% فكانت نسبتهم المئوية تتراوح بين 16% و56%. وأما مرضى السكري الذين خضعوا لفحص قاع العين خلال الاثني عشر شهراً الماضية، أو المرضى المسجَّلون المصابون بأمراض غير سارية مع تسجيلهم لضغط الدم مرتين في آخر زيارة متابعة، فكان متوسط نسبتهم المئوية 45% و40% على التوالي.

واشتملت النتائج الرئيسية المُستخلصة من هذا البحث على ضرورة تطويع المؤشرات من أجل اعتمادها في الظروف القُطرية الحالية، والتعرف على التحديات الحالية التي تعترض القياس الكامل للمؤشرات الأساسية، وضرورة اشتمال أعمال القياس المُخطَّط لها على بناء القدرات من أجل جمع البيانات واستخدامها، بما في ذلك الإشراف.

وقد أبدت بعض البلدان التزامها بقياس جودة الرعاية الصحية الأولية؛ فقد أنشأت إيران لجنة وطنية تعمل على تنفيذ الخطوات القادمة. وبدأت عُمان بالتنفيذ الميداني للمؤشرات، وقام السودان بتطويع المؤشرات، كما تم تدريب مسؤولي التنسيق في الولايات السودانية، وأضيفت بعض المؤشرات للتعبير عن الأولويات القُطرية، التي يمكن دمجها بالسياسة والاستراتيجية الوطنيتين للجودة لضمان إدراجها في الأولويات القطرية للصحة. ومنذ ذلك الحين، وافقت اللجنة الإقليمية لإقليم شرق المتوسط على قرار بشأن اعتماد مؤشرات الجودة لتحسين جودة الرعاية على مستوى الرعاية الأولية.[5]

ويُعتبر قياس الجودة خطوة حاسمة نحو تحديد المجالات الواجب تعزيزها، فضلاً عن الاستراتيجيات والتدخلات اللازمة. ويجب أن يحدث ذلك داخل البلد الواحد أو عبر بلدان متعددة من أجل اتخاذ إجراءات محلية وقياس الأداء على المستوى الإقليمي.[6] ولقد أسفر هذا العمل عن عدد من الاستنتاجات والتوصيات بشأن العمل داخل إقليم شرق المتوسط وخارجه، بما في ذلك إثبات جدوى إنشاء مجموعة مؤشرات إقليمية، وأهمية مشاركة أصحاب المصلحة، وضرورة تحسين الأعمال والتدابير الحالية مع السماح بالتطويع المحلي، وضرورة قياس الأمور المهمة، وضرورة ضمان التركيز على الناس في المؤشرات المُعدَّة.

وكان هناك عدد من التحديات التي شرعت بالفعل بعض البلدان في التصدي لها. وتشمل التوصيات الخاصة بالعمل المستقبلي: ضرورة تضمين جميع القطاعات في العمل الوطني لقياس الجودة، ضرورة التعامل مع قياس الجودة في أماكن الصراعات، ضرورة قياس الأهداف الطموحة وضمان المرونة في تغطية الأولويات عبر مجموعة متنوعة من النظم الصحية، ضرورة مواصلة العمل لتطويع أو تطوير أدوات أفضل.

المراجع

1. Donabedian A. The quality of care. How can it be assessed? *JAMA. 1988;260(12):1743–1748.*
2. Institute of Medicine (US) Committee on Quality of Health Care in America. *Crossing the Quality Chasm: A New Health System for the 21st Century.* Washington (DC): National Academies Press (US); 2001. متاح على: http://www.ncbi.nlm.nih.gov/books/NBK222274/ [جرى الاطلاع عليه في 20 آذار/مارس 2017].
3. Refinement of indicators and criteria in a quality tool for assessing quality in primary care in Canada: a Delphi Panel study. متاح على: https://pdfs.semanticscholar.org/3b92/ab32d4c42ea92e8613f467_02707ae2336fd8.pdf [جرى الاطلاع عليه في 2017/3/2].
4. Salah H and Kidd M. Family Practice in the Eastern Mediterranean Region: Universal Health Coverage and Quality Primary Care. متاح على: https://www.amazon.com/Family-Practice-Eastern-Mediterranean-SPECIAL-ebook/dp/B07K4T8TFR [جرى الاطلاع عليه في 2019/01/19].
5. المكتب الإقليمي لمنظمة الصحة العالمية لشرق المتوسط "توسيع نطاق طب الأسرة: التقدُّم المُحرز من أجل تحقيق التغطية الصحية الشاملة". متاح على: http://applications.emro.who.int/docs/RC63_Resolutions_2016_R2_19197_EN.pdf
6. WHO. Quality of care: measuring a neglected driver of improved health. متاح على: http://www.who.int/bulletin/volumes/95/6/16-180190/en/ [جرى الاطلاع عليه في 2017/02/9].

تحدي تقديم خدمات الرعاية الصحية الأولية في بلدان إقليم شرق المتوسط التي تمرُّ بأزمات

هافييه ميدول

يُعدّ إقليم شرق المتوسط لمنظمة الصحة العالمية في الوقت الحالي ساحةً لأكبر الصراعات في العالم، وقد ظل أكثر من ثلث بلدانه الأعضاء في صراع دائم طوال الفترة الماضية (ابتداءً من عام 2011 وما بعدها).

ويشمل تأثير الصراع على الصحة زيادة معدلات المراضة والوفيات بسبب العنف.[1] وأصبحت الحروب والصراعات طويلة الأمد على نحو متزايد، وأضحت تستهدف المدنيين والبنية التحتية الاجتماعية والاقتصادية، وتتسبب في نزوح جماعي للسكان الذين غالباً ما يستقرون في مناطق حضرية، بين السكان العاديين وليس في مخيمات اللاجئين أو النازحين داخلياً.[2] وغالباً ما تُسفر الفترات الطويلة للصراع المنخفض الحدة عن عدد أقل من حالات الوفاة الناجمة عن العنف، ولكن تكون لها آثار صحية أكبر على المدى الطويل، بسبب زيادة معدلات انتشار حالات الصحة النفسية، والسل، بل الأمراض غير السارية. ومن الأمور الباعثة على القلق عودة ظهور الأمراض السارية التي كان الإقليم يخلو منها منذ أكثر من عَقْد من الزمن، مثل شلل الأطفال (في سوريا والعراق) والدفتيريا (في اليمن)، مما يدل على انهيار نُظم التحصين الروتيني.[3] كما أن انهيار النظم هو السبب الجذري لانتشار وباء الكوليرا في اليمن بأبعاد لم يسبق لها مثيل.

وربما يحدّ الصراع من الوصول إلى الخدمات الصحية بأن يحدّ من قدرة النظام من خلال آليات مختلفة، منها التدمير الفعلي للمرفق الصحي، أو تعطيل سلاسل الإمداد، أو نزوح العاملين الصحيين المهرة. وأصبحت المرافق الصحية والموظفون الصحيون أهدافاً في صراعات تزداد يوماً بعد يوم.[4]

ويتأثر تنظيم خدمات الرعاية الصحية الأولية، وغيرها، بمراحل الصراع —بدءاً من إعلان الحرب وصولاً إلى إرساء السلام— أو بتنوُّع السلطات المختلفة التي تدير إقليماً كان مُوحَّداً من قبل. ويتميز الصراع المُعلَن بوجود جهات فاعلة في مجال العمل الإنساني —وهي منظمات غير حكومية في الغالب— وبإقامة نماذج متأقلمة لتوصيل الخدمات، مثل ما يُسمى "مستشفيات ميدانية" في الصراع السوري. ويُقدَّم الدعم إلى فرادى المرافق وليس النُظم، ويتقلص دور الحكومة. ويعني النزوح الجماعي أن جزءاً كبيراً من الرعاية الصحية الأولية يمكن أن يُقدَّم خارج البلد.

وقد يؤدي إرساء السلام وتحقيق الاستقرار إلى حدوث تغييرات في نموذج تقديم الخدمات، مثل التعاقد الخارجي مع منظمات غير حكومية لتقديم الخدمات في أفغانستان أو الصومال أو دارفور، أو إدراج الصحة النفسية أو التدبير العلاجي للأمراض غير السارية ضمن حزم الخدمات المُقدَّمة.

ويُروّج للحزم الأساسية للخدمات الصحية على أنها طريقة فعالة وموحدة لتوسيع نطاق تقديم الخدمات، وغالباً ما يكون ذلك في إطار عملية لإصلاح القطاع. وقد تكون هذه الحزم الأساسية خاصة بظروف إنسانية، مثل مشروع «أسفير» ومجموعة الخدمات الأولية التي تمثل الحد الأدنى. ورغم أن معظم بلدان إقليم شرق المتوسط التي تشهد صراعات قد أعدَّت حزمها الأساسية من الخدمات الصحية، فلا يكاد يوجد دليل يُذكر على تنفيذ هذه الحزم، ويُستثنى من ذلك في المقام الأول أفغانستان.

وتتزامن الأوضاع المتأزمة مع انخفاض الحيز المالي للحكومة المعنية، مما يؤدي إلى انخفاض الإنفاق الحكومي على الصحة. ويتمثل البديلان الرئيسيان في الموارد الخارجية والنفقات التي يدفعها المواطنون من أموالهم. وتشير قاعدة البيانات العالمية للإنفاق على الصحة إلى أن مستويات إنفاق المواطنين من أموالهم على الصحة تبلغ 76% من إجمالي الإنفاق على الصحة في اليمن والسودان، و64% في أفغانستان، و54% في سوريا، مقابل 20% في الأردن، و35% في تونس، و15% في المملكة العربية السعودية. وقد ثبت أن التمويل المُقدَّم من جهات مانحة له دور أساسي في مشاريع البنية التحتية/ إعادة الإعمار أو في تمويل تدخلات الإصلاح الصحي، التي غالباً ما تستجيب لأجندة خارجية.

ويتطلب تقديم توليفة الخدمات التي تشتمل على الرعاية الصحية الأولية أن تعمل التوليفة المناسبة من المهارات في المواقع المناسبة. ولكي تتمكن الفرق الأساسية من أداء واجباتها، ينبغي أن تضمن النظم الصحية القُطرية توفير الموظفين المناسبين وتوزيعهم على نحو ملائم وإدارتهم بناءً على الأداء. فبعض العوامل التي تؤثر على أداء العاملين في مجال الرعاية الصحية – مثل المعلومات والمهارات، والتحفيز، وتوفر مبادئ توجيهية سريرية مُحدَّثة، وتوفر الأجهزة والأدوية واللوازم، والتقييم الداعم – ليس من السهل الوصول إليها وإنفاذها، لا سيما في الظروف الحافلة بالتحديات. وتُعد القدرة التدريبية، وخاصةً معايير جودة التدريب، من أوائل الخسائر المُتكبَّدة في حالة الصراع. ويرتفع خلال المراحل الأولى من الأزمة معدل تناقص الكوادر العاملة في مجال الرعاية الصحية، بل يرتفع معدل هجرتهم إلى أماكن أكثر أمناً، ولكن من المهم أيضاً الاستعاضة عنهم بالعاملين في المجال الإنساني من الأجانب والمتطوعين.[5] ومما يعيق التوزيع المناسب للقوى العاملة في مجال الرعاية الصحية انعدامُ الأمن، وانخفاض الرواتب، وعدم وجود حوافز جذابة لاستبقاء الموظفين.

واتباع كثير من البلدان لنهج ممارسة طب الأسرة قد ربط هذه الاستراتيجية بوجود اختصاصي في الرعاية الصحية، واختصاصي طب الأسرة. ويؤدي ذلك إلى ظهور التحدي المزدوج المتمثل في إعداد حزمة للتدريب والاعتماد تكون جذابة لبعض من أفضل الأطباء في البلد، وإيجاد حل للأطباء الكثيرين الذين لن يحصلوا على هذا الاعتماد. وبوجد العديد من برامج طب الأسرة في بلدان إقليم شرق المتوسط، ولكنها لا تُخرج سوى عدد قليل من الاختصاصيين المعتمدين.[6]

وفي البلدان التي لا تكفل فيها النظم الرسمية الحصول على الخدمات الصحية الأساسية، يمكن تأهيل كوادر جديدة وتوظيفها وتدريبها للعمل في أبعد الأماكن وأقلها أمناً. وقد تسارعت في أفغانستان وتيرة تدريب وتوظيف قابلات مجتمعيات[7] لزيادة عدد الماهرات في التوليد بالمناطق النائية التي لا يقبل بالعمل فيها أيُّ مهني مُدرَّب من الحضر. وجرت الاستعانة بالعاملين في مجال صحة المجتمع كبديل من أجل تقديم بعض مكونات الرعاية الصحية الأولية على الأقل.

وتتطلب كل أزمة اتباع نهج مُفصل لتقديم الرعاية الصحية الأولية. أما النظم الصحية القادرة على الصمود فإنها تنهض من كبوتها مرة تلو الأخرى لتقدم أقصى ما يمكنها تقديمه من المجموعة القياسية لخدمات الرعاية الصحية الأولية. وقد يساعد وجود رؤية مستقبلية مُنَظَّمة على اجتياز العاصفة الحالية، لكن التعديل المناسب ينبغي أن يحدث كل يوم تقريباً.

المراجع

1. C. Murray, G. King, A. Lopez, N. Tomijima and E. Krug. Armed conflict as a public health problem. British Medical Journal, 2002; 324: 346-9.

2. P. Spiegel, F. Checchi, S. Colombo and E. Paik. Health-care needs of people affected by conflict: future trends and changing frameworks. Lancet, 2010; 375: 341-45.

3. R. Raslan, S. El Sayegh, S. Chams, N. Chams, A. Leone and I. Hussein. Re-emerging Vaccine-Preventable Diseases in War-Affected Peoples of the Eastern Mediterranean Region—An Update. Frontiers in Public Health, 2017; 5.

4. S. Colombo and E. Pavignani. Recurrent failings of medical humanitarianism: intractable, ignored, or just exaggerated? Lancet (online), 2017.

5. E. Pavignani. Human Resources for Health Under Stress in the Eastern Mediterranean Region. World Health Organization, 2017.

6. A. Abyad, A. Al-Baho, I. Unluoglu, M. Tarawneh and T. Al Hilfy. Development of Family Medicine in the Middle East. Family Medicine, 2007; 39 (10): 736-41.

7. X. Mòdol. Afghanistan Joint Health Sector Review and Strategic Plan Implementation Assessment. European Union, Ministry of Public Health of Afghanistan, Kabul, 2015.

شراكات بين القطاعين العام والخاص: تجربة محافظة مازندران في التعاقد مع أطباء الأسرة العاملين في القطاع الخاص، جمهورية إيران الإسلامية
محسن عربي، محسن أسدي لاري، قاسم جان بابايي

تقع محافظة مازندران في شمالي إيران على ساحل بحر قزوين، ويبلغ عدد سكانها 83.582.32 نسمة (يعيش 756.456.1 نسمة منهم في مناطق حضرية).

وبدأ برنامج طب الأسرة الريفي في المناطق الريفية بمحافظة مازندران في عام 2005، بتعيين أطباء أسرة وقابلات في المراكز الصحية الريفية لمساعدة العاملين في مجال صحة المجتمع في دُور الصحة القروية، ولتقديم حزم الخدمات الصحية لجميع الناس. وقد اكتمل نطاق التغطية بهذا البرنامج. كما يوجد نظام إحالة بين كل دار من دُور الصحة القروية ومركزها الصحي الريفي. وتُحدَّد مرتبات طبيب الأسرة والقابلة على أساس عدد المرضى.

وعلى النقيض من ذلك، لم تُقدَّم الخدمات في المرافق الصحية الحضرية. ولذلك نظر واضعو السياسات وأعضاء البرلمان في ضرورة اتباع نهج قائم على طبيب الأسرة عند تقديم الخدمات في المناطق الحضرية، وكذلك في المناطق الريفية.[1] وأُنشئت لجنة توجيهية ولجنة تنفيذية ولجنة للرصد والتقييم على مستوى المحافظات مع إشراك أصحاب المصلحة الرئيسيين.

ويتقدم إلى المركز الصحي بالمنطقة الأطباء العاملون في القطاع الخاص الذين يرغبون في العمل كأطباء أسرة في المناطق الحضرية، بدون أي ممارسة مزدوجة. كما أنهم مُلزمون بتوظيف قابلة أو ممرضة للعمل في عياداتهم. ولإبرام عقد مع مؤسسات التأمين، يُفحص الطلب المُقدَّم في الشبكة الصحية على مستوى المناطق الصحية وعلى مستوى المحافظات أيضاً. ومؤسسات التأمين هي المسؤولة عن المكافآت/المرتبات المباشرة التي يحصل عليها أطباء الأسرة بعد الموافقات الشهرية على خدماتهم المُقدَّمة. وعلى مدار السنوات الخمس الماضية، تقدم 637 طبيب أسرة بطلب في محافظة مازندران، وتعاقد أكثر من 78% منهم مع وكالات التأمين لما يزيد على ثلاث سنوات.[2]

ويبلغ عدد السكان الذين يخدمهم كل طبيب من أطباء الأسرة المتفرغين 2500 نسمة. وتُقدَّم الخدمات على مدار ثماني ساعات يومياً لضمان تحسين الحصول على الخدمات. وفي دراسة أُجريت على 1768 أسرة مُختارة عشوائياً داخل محافظة مازندران، ذُكر أن متوسط المدة الزمنية اللازمة للوصول إلى طبيب الأسرة بلغ 16.3 دقيقة سيراً على الأقدام، أو 5.6 دقائق بالسيارة.

وكانت الاستعانة بالقطاع الخاص لتقديم الخدمات إلى السكان أحد أفضل الحلول المتاحة، إذ لم تكن توجد حاجة إلى الاستثمار الحكومي في تشييد وتجهيز مرافق جديدة أو توظيف موارد بشرية إضافية. وفي بداية التعاقد، يجب أن يكون لدى الطبيب مكان مناسب، لا تقل مساحته عن 40 متراً مربعاً، فضلاً عن الأجهزة المطلوبة المذكورة في القائمة الموحدة. كما ينبغي لطبيب الأسرة أن يُعيِّن طبيباً بديلاً ليحل محله في حالة غيابه، من أجل ضمان استمرارية تقديم الرعاية. وأما في حالة أطباء الأسرة غير المتفرغين، فيلزم وجود طبيب مُناوب لنوبتي العمل الصباحية والمسائية. ويخضع أداء طبيب الأسرة للمتابعة من جانب أطباء الأسرة الآخرين وخبراء الصحة في المركز الصحي الشامل بمنطقة طبيب الأسرة. وتقوم مؤسسات التأمين والمركز الصحي للمدينة بزيارات للمتابعة الإضافية. وتُستخدم نتائج هذه المتابعة في تحديد النسبة المئوية للمكافآت التي يحصل عليها الطبيب على أساس عدد المرضى، وقد تصل هذه النسبة إلى 20% كل ثلاثة أشهر. وتقدم وزارة الصحة والتعليم الطبي حزم خدمات صحية من المستوى الأول، على أساس الفئات العمرية للسكان المشمولين بالخدمات، ويُخطر بها جميع أطباء الأسرة. وتشمل هذه الفئات العمرية حديثي الولادة، والأطفال، واليافعين، والشباب، والكُهول، وكبار السن، والأمهات الحوامل والمرضعات.

وفي دراسة أُجريت على 96 طبيباً من أطباء الأسرة في مناطق حضرية، بلغ معدل الرضا العام للأطباء المشاركين في البرنامج

3.37 من 5. وفي المقابل، أظهرت دراسة استقصائية أُجريت على 888 شخصاً في عام 2016 أن 23.8% قاموا بتغيير طبيب الأسرة مرة واحدة وأن 2.8% غيروا طبيبهم مرتين أو أكثر خلال الأشهر الاثني عشر السابقة للدراسة. وفيما يتعلق بالرضا عن الخدمات المُقدَّمة، كانت نسبة الراضين عن الخدمات 62.8% ونسبة غير الراضين عنها 37.2%.

وظهرت في أثناء تنفيذ هذا البرنامج مشاكل عديدة، منها نقص الأموال المكافئة التي تقدمها مؤسسات التأمين، عدم وجود ما يكفي من الكفاءات في صفوف أطباء الأسرة لتقديم خدمات تعزيز الصحة والوقاية الأولية، إحجام المتخصصين عن أداء دورهم وتقديم المشورة والملاحظات إلى أطباء الأسرة، التأخر في دفع المكافآت الشهرية التي يحصل عليها أطباء الأسرة على أساس عدد المرضى، انخفاض مستوى الوعي والتقبل الثقافي لخدمات طبيب الأسرة لدى السكان، التأخر في الوصول إلى السجلات الصحية الإلكترونية الفعالة.

وبعد ما يقرب من خمس سنوات من الخبرة منذ تنفيذ برنامج طبيب الأسرة الحضري في محافظة مازندران، يجري حالياً تطوير المبادرات التالية من أجل تحسين الأداء: نظام دفع كامل قائم على الأداء، مما يشجع أطباء الأسرة على العمل في مجموعات بدلاً من العمل المنفرد، رفع مستوى كفاءة أطباء الأسرة وخبراء الصحة من خلال التثقيف، استخدام نماذج تدريبية قائمة على الفرق لتعليم فرق أطباء الأسرة، الدعوة إلى الوصول إلى موارد مالية مستدامة ومكافآت منتظمة إصلاح نُظُم الدفع للأطباء المتخصصين وذوي التخصصات الفرعية.

المراجع

1. Aarabi M, Oveis G, Alaei O. Urban Family Physician in Mazandaran Province. Sary, Mazandaran (Iran): Mazandaran University of Medical Sciences and Health Services, Deputy of Public Health; 2017. Report No. 3.

2. Nasrollahpour Shirvani SD, Kabir MJ, Ashrafian Amiri H, Rabiei SM, Keshavarzi A, Farzin K. Experience of Implementing the Program of the Urban Family Physician in Iran. 1st edition. Tehran: Iran Health Organization, 2017: 93.

أفغانستان

بشير نورمال، نجيب الله صافي، شفيق الله حماد

العدد الإجمالي لمرافق الرعاية الصحية الأولية	2067
عدد الممارسين العامِّين العاملين في المرافق العامة للرعاية الصحية الأولية	2941
عدد أطباء الأسرة المعتمدين العاملين في مرافق الرعاية الصحية الأولية	70
متوسط عدد خريجي أطباء الأسرة كل سنة	8
عدد كليات الطب	37 (9 كليات حكومية، و28 كلية خاصة)
عدد أقسام طب الأسرة في كليات الطب	2

مقدمة

يتضمن النظام الصحي في أفغانستان الحزمة الأساسية للخدمات الصحية والحزمة الضرورية لخدمات المستشفيات. وتقدم الحزمة الأولى خدمات الرعاية الأولية والوقائية، في حين أن الحزمة الثانية تتألف من خدمات تُقدَّم على مستوى المستشفيات. وتوجد في مستشفيات المقاطعات عناصر كلتا الفئتين من الخدمات.

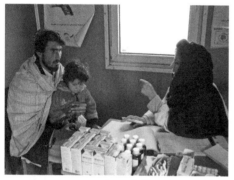

وإلى جانب هاتين الحزمتين، توجد مجموعة أخرى من المستشفيات تُسمَّى المستشفيات المتخصصة/الوطنية، وهي مراكز إحالة تُقدِّم رعاية طبية تخصصية.[1]

ويجري تمويل حزمتي الخدمات والتعاقد عليهما من خلال النظم الصحية لحكومة جمهورية أفغانستان الإسلامية، وتكون الحزمتان مصحوبتين بمساعدة تقنية يقدمها العديد من شركاء التنمية إلى وزارة الصحة العامة. وتشرف الحكومة على تقديم الخدمات الصحية، ولكن تقديمها في حد ذاته تقوم به في الغالب منظماتٌ غير حكومية. ويكاد يقتصر تمويل نظام الصحة العامة على التمويل

صيدلانية تتحدث مع مريض

المُقدَّم من موارد خارجية. وبمرور الوقت، سوف يَلزم أن تصبح الحكومة بالتدريج المموِّل الرئيسي لقطاع الصحة. وستواصل الجهات المانحة تمويل تقديم حزمتي الخدمات في جميع ولايات أفغانستان الأربعة والثلاثين حتى عام 2021.

التحديات الرئيسية

تواجه أفغانستان التحديات الخطيرة التي تواجهها أيُّ بيئة سياسية هشة، وتهديدات مستمرة من حركات التمرد وحائزي السلطة المحليين، وانكماشاً اقتصادياً، وتناقُص تدفُّقات المعونات، وانتشار الفساد، وعلاقات إقليمية لا تزال تؤدي إلى تفاقم النزاع. وقد كانت لهذه العوامل المعقدة والديناميات المرتبطة بها آثارٌ سلبية كبيرة على كفاءة الدولة وعلى جميع جوانب التنمية في أفغانستان، بما فيها قطاع الصحة. ويوجد في أفغانستان أعلى معدل خصوبة كُلي في آسيا، إذ يبلغ 5.3 مولود/امرأة، ويزداد عدد سكانها الآن بنحو مليون نسمة سنوياً.[3،4] وبوجه عام، تُعد "البنية التحتية المادية" في أفغانستان، بما فيها الطرق والإمدادات الموثوقة للمياه والطاقة، غير كافية لدعم تقديم الخدمات الصحية الموسعة والفعالة والوصول إليها. وتُعتبر الحالة الصحية للأمهات والمواليد والأطفال في أفغانستان من بين أسوأ الحالات الصحية في العالم. ويمثل سوء التغذية مشكلة خطيرة، إذ يشير تقرير صدر مؤخراً عن منظمة اليونيسف إلى أن 59% من الأطفال يعانون من التقزُّم في مرحلة الطفولة، وهي النسبة الأسوأ على مستوى العالم. وللإنفاق الشخصي نصيب كبير في النفقات الصحية في البلد، إذ تبلغ نسبة النفقات التي تدفعها الأسر من ميزانيتها 74% من مجموع النفقات.

سُبُل المضيّ قُدُماً

تتّبع وزارة الصحة العامة سبعة توجُّهات استراتيجية، ألا وهي: [1] السياسة الصحية العامة/دمج الصحة في جميع السياسات، [2] البيئة الداعمة، [3] الأعمال المجتمعية، [4] تنمية المهارات الشخصية، [5] إعادة توجيه الخدمات الصحية، [6] بناء القدرات، [7] التنسيق والشراكة.

ولوزارة الصحة العامة 10 مبادئ تشغيلية، ألا وهي: [1] التنمية الخاضعة لسيطرة الدولة وتوجيهها، [2] الحوكمة الرشيدة، بما في ذلك الشفافية الفعالة والمساءلة،[1] [3] الحق في الصحة للجميع، لا سيما للنساء والأطفال وأفراد الفئات الضعيفة، [4] التوازن بين الجنسين، [5] تعزيز مَواطن القوة من خلال الشراكات الداخلية والخارجية والتنسيق، [6] المساهمة والمشاركة المجتمعية الفعالة، [7] ثقافة الاعتماد على الأدلة عند التخطيط واتخاذ القرارات، والتوجه نحو النتائج، والإدارة القائمة على النتائج، [8] تعزيز "التفكير المنظومي" على جميع المستويات، [9] ثقافة التآزر والعمل الجماعي المتعدد المهام، [10] التركيز على تعزيز الصحة والوقاية.[2]

وقد أسفر تحسين إتاحة الخدمات وتوسيع نطاق التغطية عن بعض النتائج الباهرة، حيث انخفض معدل وفيات الرضع من 66 حالة وفاة لكل 1000 ولادة حيَّة في عام 2005 إلى 45 حالة وفاة في عام 2017. وخلال الفترة نفسها، انخفض معدل وفيات الأطفال حديثي الولادة من 31 إلى 22، وانخفض معدل وفيات الأطفال دون سن الخامسة من 87 إلى 55 لكل 1000 ولادة حيَّة، وارتفعت نسبة القابلات الماهرات من 14% في عام 2003 إلى أكثر من 50% في عام 2017.[4] وحدث أيضاً انخفاض شديد في معدل وفيات الأمهات، إذ انخفض من 1600 وفاة إلى 396 وفاة لكل 100 ألف ولادة حية.[3] وشهدت أيضاً مؤشرات التغطية بالخدمات الأساسية الخاصة بصحة الأمهات والأطفال زيادة كبيرة، إذ ارتفعت التغطية بخدمات الرعاية السابقة للولادة من 16% إلى 59%، وارتفع معدل انتشار وسائل منع الحمل من 10% إلى 23%، وزادت نسبة الولادة في المؤسسات الصحية من أقل من 15% إلى 48%، وزادت التغطية بالجرعة الثالثة من اللقاح الثلاثي/الخماسي للأطفال من سن يوم واحد إلى 23 شهراً من 30% إلى 58%.[4]

المراجع

1. Essential Package of Health Services for Afghanistan, 2005.
2. Ministry of Public Health. *Afghanistan Health Indicators Fact Sheet.* 2014. متاح على:
http://moph.gov.af/Content/Media/Documents/AfghanistanHealthIndicatorsFactsheetFeb20146122014102616511553325325.pdf
[جرى الاطلاع عليه في 31 كانون الثاني/يناير 2018].
3. Central Statistics Organization (CSO), Ministry of Public Health (MoPH), and ICF. *Afghanistan Demographic and Health Survey 2015.* Kabul, Afghanistan, and Rockville, Maryland, USA. 2017.
4. *Central Statistics Organization.* National Risk and Vulnerability Assessment 2011–12. Afghanistan Living Condition Survey. *Kabul, CSO. 2012.*

البحرين
فيصل عبد اللطيف الناصر، عادل الصياد

العدد الإجمالي لمرافق الرعاية الصحية الأولية	28
عدد الممارسين العامّين العاملين في المرافق العامة للرعاية الصحية الأولية	98
عدد أطباء الأسرة المعتمدين العاملين في مرافق الرعاية الصحية الأولية	228
متوسط عدد خريجي أطباء الأسرة كل سنة	22
عدد كليات الطب	2
عدد أقسام طب الأسرة	1

مقدمة

حقَّقت البحرين الأهداف الإنمائية للألفية التي حددتها الأمم المتحدة في قطاع الصحة، وذلك قبل خمس سنوات من الموعد المُتفق عليه وهو عام 2015.[1] وارتفع متوسط العمر المتوقع في مملكة البحرين ارتفاعاً كبيراً، فبلغ 77.2 سنة في عام 2015 مقابل 73.4 سنة في عام 2000.[2] وأدى ذلك إلى زيادة عدد السكان كبار السن الذين تزيد احتياجاتهم من الرعاية الصحية.[3]

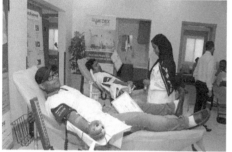

مرفق رعاية صحية أولية في البحرين

وتوجد في مراكز الرعاية الصحية الأولية بالمملكة معظم المرافق والخدمات الأساسية، بما فيها طب الأسرة. ولا يُسجَّل في أي مركز صحي سوى المُقيمين في نطاقه الجغرافي، ولا يُسمح لهؤلاء باستشارة مراكز صحية أخرى دون إحالة. وتخضع الخدمات العلاجية والوقائية التي تُقدِّمها المراكز لإشراف مباشر من أطباء الأسرة. وغالباً ما يُخصَّص لكل أسرة طبيب مُحدَّد (أيْ طبيبها الخاص المتخصص في طب الأسرة). وفي الآونة الأخيرة، بدأ استخدام سجلات طبية إلكترونية (النظام الوطني للمعلومات الصحية (I-Seha)) حيث تُحفظ بيانات المريض في خادوم ويمكن أن تطلع عليها، بعد الحصول على موافقة المريض، شتى أقسام النظام الصحي مثل أقسام الرعاية الثانوية والرعاية التخصصية وغيرها من المرافق الصحية.

وتُقدَّم خدمة الرعاية الصحية الأولية مجاناً للبحرينيين، ومقابل رسوم للوافدين إذا كانوا غير مشمولين بتأمين صحي. ويوجد في مرافق الرعاية الصحية الأولية نظام جيد لإحالة المرضى إلى الرعاية الثانوية إذا احتاج المريض إلى مزيد من الفحص أو العلاج أو إلى استشارة طبيب آخر. وتُرسَل فيما بعدُ جميع المعلومات إلى الطبيب الذي أحال المريض.

بدأ برنامج طب الأسرة في عام 1979، وكان حدثاً فارقاً في تحسين قطاع الصحة. ويرجع كل الفضل إلى القرار الشجاع الذي اتخذه السياسي الدكتور علي فخرو، وزير الصحة الأسبق، الذي كان من أشد المؤمنين بطب الأسرة ومن أقوى المؤيدين له، وكانت لديه رؤية صحية ثبت أنها الرؤية المناسبة للبحرين.

التحديات الرئيسية

رغم أن البحرين كانت أول دولة في منطقة الخليج تبدأ برنامج الإقامة الطبية في طب الأسرة وتُقدم خدمات الرعاية الصحية الأولية لسكانها، فإنها تواجه العديد من التحديات التي قد تمنعها من تطبيق الخدمات الكاملة لطب الأسرة. وتتمثل إحدى أهم العقبات في قلة عدد الأطباء المتخصصين في طب الأسرة حتى الآن، فهو أقل بكثير من العدد المطلوب. فالبحرين، بتعدادها السكاني الحالي، تحتاج إلى 696 طبيباً من أطباء الأسرة المُدرَّبين تدريباً جيداً، في حين أن القوة العاملة المتوفرة نصف هذا

العدد تقريباً، مما يعني وجود طبيب أسرة واحدة لكل 3580 نسمة وهو ما يقل بكثير عن النسبة المُثلى. أما التحدي الخطير الآخر، الذي يتعلق أيضاً بنقص عدد أطباء الأسرة، فهو أن عبء المرضى المُلقى على عاتق أطباء الأسرة المؤهلين تمامَ التأهيل يفوق طاقاتهم، مما يمنحهم وقتاً أقل لتطبيق الممارسة المثالية لطب الأسرة.

سُبُل المضيّ قُدُماً

للتغلب على تلك التحديات، يجب أن يعتمد واضعو السياسات استراتيجية حازمة تنص على ما يلي:

- ينبغي أن تتبع الحكومة استراتيجية واضحة تَعتبر طبَّ الأسرة والرعاية الصحية الأولية أساساً للنظام الصحي في المملكة.

- ينبغي زيادة ميزانية الرعاية الصحية المُخصَّصة لخدمات الرعاية الصحية الأولية، على غرار الميزانية المُخصَّصة لخدمات الرعاية الثانوية والتخصصية.

- علاوة على ذلك، يجب اتخاذ قرار شجاع لزيادة عدد أطباء الأسرة المتخصصين من خلال زيادة عدد برامج الأطباء المقيمين ليوجد أكثر من برنامج واحد، وزيادة قدرة البرنامج الحالي على استيعاب أكثر من ثلاثين طبيباً سنوياً. فالمعدل الحالي لتخرُّج أطباء الأسرة الذي يبلغ 16 طبيباً جديداً كل عام يعني أن تخرُّج العدد الذي تحتاج إليه المملكة من أطباء الأسرة سيستغرق 22 عاماً على الأقل.

المراجع

1. الرعاية الصحية في البحرين. http://www.bahrain.com/en/bi/key-investment-sectors/Pages/Healthcare.aspx#.WfrUAztx3cs [جرى الاطلاع عليه في 22 أيلول/سبتمبر 2018].

2. إحصاءات وزارة الصحة لعام 2015. https://www.moh.gov.bh/Content/Files/Publications/statistics/HS2015/hs2015_e.htm [جرى الاطلاع عليها في 22 أيلول/سبتمبر 2018].

3. Alnasir Faisal "Ageing and Pattern of Population Changes in the Developing Countries". **The Middle East Journal of Age & Aging. 2015: 12:2; 26–32.**

جيبوتي
عبدولاي كوناتي

العدد الإجمالي لمرافق الرعاية الصحية الأولية	71
عدد الممارسين العامّين العاملين في المؤسسات العامة للرعاية الصحية الأولية	51
عدد أطباء الأسرة المعتمدين العاملين في مؤسسات الرعاية الصحية الأولية	صفر
متوسط عدد خريجي طب الأسرة في السنة	صفر
عدد كليات الطب	1
عدد أقسام طب الأسرة	صفر

مقدمة

كثَّفت الحكومة جهودها الرامية إلى زيادة عدد مرافق الرعاية الصحية الأولية، لا سيما المراكز الصحية الفرعية التي زاد عددها من 22 في عام 2004 إلى 38 في عام 2016، بزيادة نسبتها 73%. وخلال الفترة نفسها، ارتفع عدد المراكز الصحية من 8 مراكز إلى 15 مركزاً، بزيادة نسبتها 88%. وإضافةً إلى القطاع شبه العام، توجد 10 مرافق للرعاية الصحية الأولية. ولم يُعتمد بعدُ تطبيق طب الأسرة وممارسته في جيبوتي. وبهدف تعزيز القطاع الوقائي، أنشأت الحكومة المعهد الوطني للصحة العامة في جيبوتي، ومرافق للمجالات الصحية ذات الأولوية مثل صحة الأمهات والأطفال، والتحصين، والملاريا، والسل، وفيروس نقص المناعة البشرية، بالإضافة إلى توفير الرعاية العلاجية. وقد ساعدت هذه المبادرات الحكومية جميعها على تحسين وضع الرعاية الصحية الأولية في جيبوتي، رغم أنه لا يزال لازماً بذلُ مزيد من الجهود لتقليل عبء المرض المُلقى على كاهل السكان.

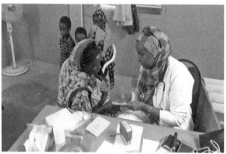

طبيبة مع مريضة في أحد مرافق الرعاية الصحية الأولية

وقد شهدت صحة الأمهات والأطفال تحسناً، حيث انخفض معدل وفيات الأمهات لكل 100 ألف ولادة حيَّة من 740 في عام 1996 إلى 383 في عام 2012، أي بانخفاض قدره 50% تقريباً. وبين عامي 2002 و2012، انخفض معدل وفيات الرضع والأطفال من 131 إلى 68 لكل 1000 ولادة حيَّة، وانخفض معدل وفيات الرضع من 108 إلى 68 لكل 1000 ولادة حيَّة، وانخفض معدل وفيات الأطفال حديثي الولادة من 45 إلى 36 لكل 1000 ولادة حيَّة.[1] وكان معدل انتشار مرض السل 906 حالات لكل 100 ألف نسمة في عام 2014. وانخفض معدل الإصابة من 619 حالة جديدة لكل 100 ألف نسمة في عام 2013 إلى 378 حالة جديدة في عام 2015. وعلى الرغم من هذا الاتجاه التنازلي، لا تزال جيبوتي بها أحد أعلى معدلات الإصابة بمرض السل في العالم. ولا يزال تكامل الخدمات الصحية الأساسية إحدى أولويات حكومة جيبوتي منذ سنوات عديدة.[2]

وقد حددت الخريطة الصحية للبلد، التي وُضعت في عام 2006، مجموعة دنيا من الخدمات المتكاملة. ويوجد نظام إحالة وإحالة مرتدة بين شتى مستويات الهرم الصحي، وهذا النظام يُسهِّل على المرضى الدخول المباشر إلى المستشفيات، كما أن العلاج مجاني. ولكن عمليات التحويل والإحالة في حالة البالغين ليست على القدر الجيد نفسه من التنظيم، وليست مجانية. ووفقاً لاستراتيجية الرعاية الصحية الأولية، يوفِّر النظام الصحي منذ عام 2003 الأدوية الجنيسة الأساسية، التي جرى تحديثها في عام 2016. وقد شهدت الموارد البشرية الصحية زيادة كبيرة. ففي عام 2016، بلغ عدد الممارسين العامّين 1.06 لكل 10000 نسمة، وبلغ عدد المساعدين الطبيين 8.18 لكل 10000 نسمة.[3] وارتفع عدد العاملين في مجال الرعاية الصحية من 1664 عام 2008 إلى 3381 عام 2017، أيْ بنسبة زيادة تفوق 100%.

التحديات الرئيسية

وفقاً لنتائج تقييم توفر الخدمات والتأهب لعام 2015، يبلغ مؤشر توفر البنى التحتية الصحية على الصعيد الوطني 38.9%. وفي الواقع، لم يصل ثلثا أقاليم البلد إلى المتوسط الوطني. ولم تُجرَ أي دراسات لتوضيح معدل انتشار الأمراض غير السارية ومعدل الإصابة بها وأنماطها. وتتسبب الأمراض غير السارية في 40% من حالات دخول المستشفى، وفي ثلث حالات الوفاة في مستشفى بلتيير العام في مدينة جيبوتي. وما زالت جيبوتي تفتقر إلى برنامج جودة واعتماد لخدماتها الصحية. ولا توجد بروتوكولات منسقة على الصعيد الوطني بشأن معظم الأمراض. ويلزم بذل جهود لتحقيق التكامل في الرعاية الصحية الأولية والتحري عن الأمراض غير السارية وعلاجها ورصدها. كما أن 43% من وفيات الأطفال دون سن الخامسة في جيبوتي ترجع إلى سوء التغذية. وفيما يخص التمويل الصحي، تكمن التحديات في الحاجة إلى زيادة الميزانية المُخصَّصة للرعاية الصحية من الميزانية العامة، وجذْب تمويلات من مصادر خارجية، وتوسيع نطاق التأمين الصحي الشامل.

سُبُل المضيّ قُدُماً

لتحسين جودة خدمات الرعاية الصحية الأولية، يجب اتخاذ الإجراءات التالية: [1] تطوير أنشطة صحة المجتمع، [2] تكييف الرعاية الصحية لتلبية احتياجات المرضى، [3] توسيع نطاق اتباع نهج عالي الجودة ليشمل المستشفيات والمراكز المتخصصة، [4] ضمان استمرارية الرعاية بين المستويات المختلفة، ابتداءً من المجتمع المحلي فصاعداً، [5] تحسين تأهب النظام الصحي لإدارة تدفقات الهجرة والأزمات الإنسانية، [6] زيادة حصول سكان المناطق الريفية والنائية على الرعاية الصحية، [7] إعداد استراتيجية متكاملة لتعزيز الصحة، [8] تحديث حزمة الأنشطة الدنيا، مع التركيز على تكامل الخدمات، لا سيما فيما يخص الأمراض غير السارية، [9] إقامة شراكات وعلاقات تعاقدية، [10] رسم خريطة طريق للإصلاح الشامل لنظام المعلومات الصحية، [11] وضع خطة استراتيجية لتنمية الموارد البشرية.

المراجع

1. التقرير الختامي للدراسة الاستقصائية، المشروع العربي لإجراء دراسة استقصائية بشأن صحة الأسرة، جيبوتي. 2012.
2. الإحصاءات الصحية الوطنية. جيبوتي. 2016.
3. التقرير السنوي لإدارة الموارد المالية والبشرية، جيبوتي. 2017.

مصر

أميمة الجبالي، مجدي بكر، منى حافظ محمود الناقة، تغريد محمد فرحات، نجوى نشأت حجازي

5391	العدد الإجمالي لمرافق الرعاية الصحية الأولية
14973	عدد الممارسين العامّين العاملين في المرافق العامة للرعاية الصحية الأولية
256	عدد أطباء الأسرة المعتمدين العاملين في مرافق الرعاية الصحية الأولية
180	متوسط عدد خريجي أطباء الأسرة كل سنة
29	عدد كليات الطب
8	عدد أقسام طب الأسرة

مقدمة

بدأت ممارسة طب الأسرة في مصر في عام 1999 كاستراتيجية من استراتيجيات برنامج إصلاح قطاع الصحة، وكانت تتخذ شكل نهج متكامل لتقديم الخدمات الصحية الأساسية، وكانت تُسمى في الغالب "نموذج صحة الأسرة".[1] وكان هذا النموذج، وفقاً لتصميمه الأصلي، نهجاً متكاملاً لزيادة النطاق الجغرافي للخدمات الأساسية المُقدمة للأسر، بما فيها التدخلات الصحية والسكانية. فكل طبيب أسرة، بمساعدة فريق صحي متعدد التخصصات، يخدم الأسر الموجودة داخل نطاق المرفق الصحي، التي يتراوح عددها بين 5000 و10000 أسرة.

وكان إعداد حزمة الخدمات الأساسية التي يلزم تقديمها إلى جميع سكان مصر عنصراً رئيسياً من عناصر برنامج إصلاح قطاع الصحة الذي بدأ في عام 1997 – والتي كانت تُسمّى "حزمة المستحقات الأساسية".

توعية مجتمعية من خلال نموذج صحة الأسرة

وكان تحسين جودة الخدمات أحد الأهداف الرئيسية لبرنامج إصلاح قطاع الصحة في مصر. وفي إطار استراتيجيات البرنامج، أُنشئت "إدارة تحسين الجودة" بموجب القرار الوزاري رقم 272 لسنة 1998. ووضعت إدارة الجودة برنامجاً شاملاً لتحسين الجودة من خلال تصميم وتطبيق نظام اعتماد. وفي تموز/يوليو 2007، اعتمدت الجمعية الدولية لجودة الرعاية الصحية (ISQua) معايير الاعتماد المصرية للمستشفيات والرعاية في العيادات الخارجية والرعاية الصحية الأولية، فكانت مصر أول دولة في الإقليم تحصل على هذه الشهادة.[2]

ويُعتبر تنفيذ نموذج صحة الأسرة في مصر وتطويره مساهمة قوية في التغطية الصحية الشاملة، لأنه يستلزم تقديم خدمات متكاملة وجيدة لجميع السكان ويراعي رفاهيتهم النفسية والاجتماعية، إلى جانب آليات الحماية الاجتماعية المُحددة جيداً، حيث تتولى الدولة تلبية احتياجات الرعاية الصحية للفقراء وأفراد الفئات السكانية الضعيفة.[3]

التحديات الرئيسية

- في ظل تفكُّك النظام الصحي بأكمله، يوجد تفكُّك في الأطر المؤسسية والتنظيمية.

- ضمان وجود فرق صحية كافية ومدرَّبة ومتحمسة وتتمتع بمستوى تعليمي رفيع وتحصل على أجور مجزية في مرافق صحة الأسرة.

- يتكرر حدوث نقص في الأدوية اللازمة لدعم حزمة الخدمات.

- تعاني إدارة المعلومات من استخدام سجلات يدوية، والتجزُّؤ، والازدواجية، وتباطؤ الأتمتة، فضلاً عن ضعف تبادل المعلومات واستخدامها.
- نظام إحالة مختلّ يفتقر إلى ترتيبات مؤسسية.
- المشاركة المجتمعية "نظرية" نوعاً ما.

سُبُل المضيّ قُدُماً

- **الترتيبات المؤسسية والتنظيمية: تنقيح وتحديث وتوحيد الأطر المؤسسية والتنظيمية والمالية لنموذج صحة الأسرة.**
- حل أو تصحيح المسائل المتعلقة بالخدمة الإلزامية لخريجي كليات الطب (التي تُسمى "التكليف").
- ترشيد السجلات الطبية والتسجيل، مع تجنب الازدواجية والتدفق المتعدد.
- إعداد حزمة خدمات جيدة التوازن من خلال التحليل المنهجي لعبء المرض ودراسات تقدير التكاليف.
- وضع وتنفيذ ترتيبات مؤسسية مُحكمة تقضي بالإحالة للحصول على خدمات مُحدَّدة بوضوح.
- تنفيذ الشراء الاستراتيجي لخدمات صحة الأسرة من خلال عقود مع آليات السداد المناسبة لمُقدمي الخدمات كطريقة فعالة لتحسين أداء مُقدمي الخدمات.
- تعزيز دور المجتمع من خلال تعزيز المبادرات المجتمعية.

المراجع

1. Lie DA, Boker JR, Lenahan PM, Dow E, Scherger, JE. An international physician education program to support the recent introduction of family medicine in Egypt. *Family Medicine, 2004; 36(10): 739–746.*
2. Roadmap to achieve social justice in health care in Egypt. *World Bank.* 2015.
3. Devi S. Universal health coverage law approved in Egypt. *Lancet, 2018; 391(10117): 194.* متاح على: https://www.thelancet.com/journals/lancet/article/PIIS0140–6736(18)30091–6/fulltext [جرى الاطلاع عليه في 22 أيلول/سبتمبر 2018].

جمهورية إيران الإسلامية
محمد رضا رهبر، علي رضا رئيسي، محسن أسدي-لاري، هاستي سنائي-شوار

27173	العدد الإجمالي لمرافق الرعاية الصحية الأولية
9500	عدد الممارسين العاّمين العاملين في المرافق العامة للرعاية الصحية الأولية
66	عدد جامعات العلوم الطبية (الحكومية)
85	عدد كليات الطب
1000	عدد الممارسين العاّمين الحاصلين على ماجستير طب الأسرة (مدة الدراسة سنتان)
86	عدد اختصاصيي طب الأسرة
174	عدد أطباء الأسرة المقيمين

مقدمة

إن شتى الخطط والمشاريع التي شهدتها العقود الأربعة الماضية قد حدّدت معالم شبكة الرعاية الأولية الصحية الحالية وتوجُّهها الحالي نحو ممارسة طب الأسرة وتحقيق التغطية الصحية الشاملة. ويمكن تقسيم عملية تشكيل الشبكة الصحية الحالية إلى ثلاث مراحل.

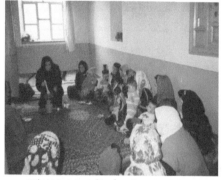

إحدى العاملات في مجال صحة المجتمع تُدرّب الأمهات على طبي الطعام لأطفالهن

انطوت المرحلة الأولى على تطوير شبكة الرعاية الصحية الأولية. وكانت السياسات الأساسية لهذه المرحلة تتمثل في تقديم الوقاية على العلاج، وتقديم المناطق الريفية النائية والمحرومة على المناطق الحضرية، وأخيراً تقديم خدمات العيادات الخارجية على خدمات المرضى الداخليين. وكان مشروع أذربيجان الغربية، الذي بدأ في عام 1971، أحد أهم التدابير التي أدت إلى بدء هذه المرحلة.[1] وبدأ منذ عام 1984 إنشاء شبكة الرعاية الصحية الأولية على نطاق واسع، وعلى مدى عشر سنوات، اتسع نطاق التغطية بخدمات الرعاية الصحية الأولية فشمل 90% من سكان الريف.[2] وفي عام 2019، شملت خدمات الرعاية الصحية الأولية أكثر من 98% من سكان الريف من خلال 17884 داراً من دُور الصحة في المستوى الأول من تقديم الخدمات و2644 مركزاً صحياً ريفياً في المستوى الثاني من الرعاية. وتُقدَّم الخدمات نفسها تقريباً إلى المجتمعات الحضرية، من خلال 4111 مركزاً صحياً فرعياً في المستوى الأول و2534 مركزاً صحياً حضرياً في المستوى الثاني. وتُحدِّد الخطة الرئيسية أين ينبغي أن تقع المرافق.[3] ويتولى تشغيلَ دُور الصحة العاملون في مجال صحة المجتمع (بهفارتس) الذين يؤدون مهام متعددة ويجتازون دورة تدريبية تتعلق بهذه المهام.[4] **ويعمل في المراكز الصحية الفرعية** خبراء مختلفون في مجال الرعاية الصحية. ويعمل في المراكز الصحية الريفية والحضرية ممارسون عامُّون وتقنيون صحيون وموظفون إداريون.[5]

وانطوت المرحلة الثانية على تطوير ممارسة طب الأسرة في المناطق الريفية وفي المدن التي يقل عدد سكانها عن 20 ألف نسمة. وبدأت هذه المرحلة بقرار برلماني صدر في عام 2005، من أجل وضع تشريع يُنظم ممارسة طب الأسرة. وأُلزمت هيئة التأمين الصحي بإصدار بطاقات تأمين صحي لجميع سكان المناطق الريفية والمجتمعات الحضرية التي يقل عدد سكانها عن 20 ألف نسمة. وكان يجب تنفيذ هذه الخدمات في إطار ممارسة طب الأسرة ونظام الإحالة.[6] وشرعت الفرق الصحية، التي انضم إليها أعضاء جدد، في تقديم خدمات جديدة في المراكز الصحية التي كانت حينذاك تُسمى مراكز الخدمات الصحية الشاملة.[7] وأُعِدَّت برامج متنوعة لتعزيز قدرة أطباء الأسرة، وكذلك أعضاء الفريق الصحي، بما في ذلك مراجعة المنهج

الدراسي للعاملين في مجال الصحة، ودورة افتراضية مقسمة إلى وحدات دراسية لماجستير طب الأسرة [8]، وبرنامج تخصُّصي في طب الأسرة.

وكانت المرحلة الثالثة هي تطوير ممارسة طب الأسرة في المدن التي يزيد عدد سكانها عن 20 ألف نسمة. وتستهدف هذه المرحلة من البرنامج السكان الذين يعيشون في مناطق حضرية، ومنهم السكان المهمَّشون حول المدن، والمدن التي يقطنها أكثر من 20 ألف نسمة. ويهدف البرنامج إلى تحقيق التغطية الصحية الشاملة في جميع أنحاء البلد. ويعتمد هذا البرنامج على إقامة شراكات بين القطاعين العام والخاص، وتفويض القطاع غير الحكومي في تقديم الخدمات.

التحديات

يتمثل التحدي الرئيسي الذي يواجه النظام الصحي الإيراني في التحول السكاني، بسبب زيادة عدد السكان المسنين الذين تزداد إصابتهم بالأمراض غير السارية، وزيادة النفقات الصحية، ومحدودية الموارد. ويتمثل التحدي الثاني في زيادة التهميش، وعدم وجود تغطية صحية كافية في المناطق المهمشة. وتشمل التحديات الأخرى الظروف التي تؤدي إلى إخفاق السوق الصحية، واختلالات في نظام الإحالة.

سُبُل المضيّ قُدُماً

تشمل سبل المضي قدماً تحسين تنظيم السوق الصحية من خلال تطوير ممارسة طب الأسرة ونظام الإحالة، وتحسين التمويل المستدام والدعم المالي للمرضى، وتحسين الجودة وزيادة نطاق التغطية بالخدمات الصحية، وإقامة شراكات اجتماعية، وتقديم رعاية صحية محورها الناس مع التعاون بين القطاعات، ووضع خطط للسيطرة على عوامل الخطر الصحية، ومعالجة المُحدِّدات الاجتماعية للصحة.

المراجع

1. King M. An Iranian Experiment in Primary Health Care: The West Azerbaijan Project. *New York: Oxford University Press; 1983.*
2. Shadpour K. *The PHC Experience in Iran.* Tehran: UNICEF; 1994.
3. Pileroudi C. The District Primary Health Care Networks in Iran. *2nd ed. Tehran: UNICEF; 1999.*
4. Rahbar MR, Ahmadi M. Lessons learnt from the model of instructional system for training community health workers in Rural HHs of Iran. *Iran Red Crescent Medical Journal.* 2015;17(2): e2145.
5. Ministry of Health and Medical Education (MoHME). *Health Network Standards.* 2017.
6. MoHME. Evaluation Study of Family Physician Programme in Rural Areas and Cities under 20 Thousand Population. *Tehran: Noavaran Sina Press; 2013.*
7. MoHME. Executive Order for Family Practice and Rural Health Insurance. 2017.
8. Ministry of Health and Medical Education of Iran. *Educational programme of Master of Family Medicine for General Practitioners.* Approved 2008.

العراق
عبد المنعم الدباغ، غيث صبري محمد، ثامر الحلفي

2600	العدد الإجمالي لمرافق الرعاية الصحية الأولية
*2362	عدد الممارسين العامّين العاملين في المرافق العامة للرعاية الصحية الأولية
350	عدد أطباء الأسرة المعتمدين العاملين في مرافق الرعاية الصحية الأولية
80–90	متوسط عدد خريجي أطباء الأسرة كل سنة
27	عدد كليّات الطب
27	عدد أقسام طب الأسرة

* باستثناء إقليم كردستان.

مقدمة

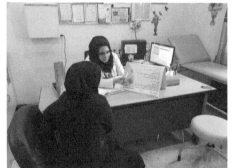
الرعاية السابقة للولادة

ترکّز اهتمام معظم الجهات المانحة المعنية بإعادة بناء الخدمات الصحية في العراق، عقب الغزو الذي وقع في عام 2003، على مشاكل المستشفيات. وشهدت السنوات العشر الماضية بالأخصّ اهتماماً بخدمات الرعاية الصحية الأولية.[1] وتتكامل حزم الخدمات الصحية الأساسية تكاملاً جيداً على مستوى مراكز الرعاية الصحية الرئيسية التي يُديرها في الغالب ممارسون مُدرَّبون تدريباً جيداً وفي بعض الحالات أطباء أسرة معتمدون، ولكن هذه الخدمات ليست على قدر جيد من التكامل على مستوى المراكز الصحية الفرعية التي يُديرها مساعدون طبيون تتمثل مهمتهم الوحيدة في إدارة حالات الطوارئ الحادة.

ويوجد 230 مركزاً من مراكز الرعاية الصحية التي تتَّبع نموذج طب الأسرة وتحتفظ منذ عهد بعيد بملفات أسرية وبها أنظمة إحالة وبرامج تدريبية مستمرة.[2] وقد اختارت منظمة الصحة العالمية تسعة مراكز لتتبُّع نهج ممارسة طب الأسرة، وتستخدم هذه المراكز التسعة نظاماً إلكترونياً للمعلومات الصحية، وتخضع لإجراءات صارمة لضمان الجودة والاعتماد. ويسود الرضا عن خدمات الرعاية الصحية الأولية، ولا يوجد اختلاف ملحوظ في المستويات بين القطاعين العام والخاص. ويُفضِّل السكان الأكثر فقراً خدمات مراكز الرعاية الصحية الأولية التابعة للقطاع العام، ويعتبرونها من أهم الجهات المُقدِّمة للخدمات الصحية. وتُقدَّم خدمات مراكز الرعاية الصحية الأولية بالمجان، ولا توجد أدلة تُذكر على دفع مبالغ مالية بصفة غير رسمية إلى مُقدمي الخدمات.[3]

وترتبط ممارسة طب الأسرة بمبادرات أخرى مثل المستشفيات ومتخصصي الرعاية الثانوية من خلال قنوات كثيرة مثل: [1] نظام الإحالة الذي يتواصل فيه أطباء الأسرة مع أطباء المستشفيات (أطباء الرعاية الثانوية) ويتلقون منهم التعقيبات ويتعاونون على تكييف التدبير العلاجي لمرضاهم، [2] برنامج زمالة تدريبي لطلاب طب الأسرة في بعض المستشفيات التعليمية، [3] أنشطة علمية مشتركة متكررة تُجرى في إطار البرامج التدريبية لمراكز صحة الأسرة، مع دعوة أطباء الرعاية الثانوية لمناقشة أحدث التطورات والمستجدات في تخصصاتهم.

التحديات الرئيسية

يمكن تلخيص التحديات الرئيسية التي تواجه ممارسة طب الأسرة فيما يلي:[4، 5]

1. تدفع الحكومة أجوراً متساوية للعاملين الصحيين بغض النظر عن اختلاف عبء العمل، مما يخلق لدى العاملين الصحيين شعوراً بعدم الإنصاف.

2. توجد فجوة كبيرة بين التمويل الحكومي المتاح وما هو مطلوب.

3. ضعف الوعي المجتمعي بطب الأسرة.

4. لا يوجد دافع قوي يحفز الأطباء المبتدئين والممارسين العامّين على التخصص في طب الأسرة.

سُبُل المضيّ قُدُماً

فيما يلي مثالان ناجحان على تطبيق المرافق الصحية لممارسة طب الأسرة:

- زيادة معدل التغطية بالتطعيم ليصل إلى 98% من المُستهدَفين، كما حدث بمركز باب المعظم لصحة الأسرة على سبيل المثال.

- زيادة عدد الأشخاص الذين يخضعون لفحص ارتفاع ضغط الدم والسكري، من أجل إشراك جميع المُستهدَفين تقريباً.

وتدعم وزارة الصحة التوسع في ممارسة طب الأسرة من خلال زيادة عدد مراكز الرعاية الأولية باستخدام نهج ممارسة طب الأسرة، وزيادة عدد أطباء الأسرة بعد التدريب الأكاديمي. وتتمثل أسباب قلة عدد أطباء الأسرة في العراق فيما يلي: [1] لا يوجد سوى برنامج إقامة واحد في مجال طب الأسرة، ولا يستطيع هذا البرنامج تخريج أكثر مما يتراوح بين 30 و 40 مرشحاً في السنة. ولم يتجاوز عدد أطباء الأسرة المعتمدين الذين تخرجوا في هذا البرنامج 200 مرشح منذ أن بدأ البرنامج في عام 1995. [2] يبلغ عدد خريجي برنامج الإقامة الخاص بالمجلس العربي في العراق، منذ عام 2008، 150 خريجاً. [3] أدت الهجرة خارج الوطن و"نزوح ذوي الكفاءات" إلى زيادة العجز في عدد أطباء الأسرة المتاحين.

المراجع

1. وزارة الصحة، حكومة العراق. النظم الصحية القائمة على الرعاية الصحية الأولية في العراق. المؤتمر الدولي المعني بالرعاية الصحية الأولية. 2008. الدوحة، قطر.

2. وزارة الصحة، حكومة العراق، المدير العام للصحة العامة. مراسلة شخصية.

3. Burnham G, et al. Perceptions and utilization of primary health care services in Iraq: findings from a national household survey. BMC International Health and Human Rights, 2011; 11: 15. متاح على: https://bmcinthealthhumrights.biomedcentral.com/articles/10.1186/1472-698X-11-15.

4. Ahmed SM. Expectations of physicians working in Erbil city about the role of family medicine practice. WONCA World Conference. Prague. 2013.

5. Issa S. Family doctors' satisfaction: a sample from Baghdad. Iraqi Postgraduate Medical Journal, 2016; 109 (3): 15–18.

الأردن

عريب الصمادي، محمد رسول الطراونة، مي هاني الحديدي

الأونروا	الجامعات	الخدمات الطبية الملكية	وزارة الصحة	
25	4	12	الشاملة: 102	العدد الإجمالي لمرافق الرعاية الصحية
			الأولية: 377	
			القروية: 187	
صفر	5–4 منذ 1999	3–2 منذ 1985	20 منذ 1993	متوسط عدد خريجي أطباء الأسرة كل سنة
			1645	عدد الممارسين العامّين العاملين في المرافق العامة للرعاية الصحية الأولية
			115 (الإجمالي: 210 أطباء يعملون في وزارة الصحة)	عدد أطباء الأسرة المعتمدين العاملين في مرافق الرعاية الصحية الأولية
			6	عدد كليات الطب
			3	عدد أقسام طب الأسرة

الأونروا: وكالة الأمم المتحدة لإغاثة وتشغيل اللاجئين الفلسطينيين في الشرق الأدنى

مقدمة

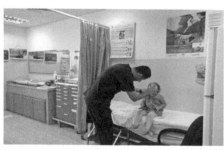
طبيب يفحص طفلة مريضة

تسعى الحكومة إلى توفير تغطية صحية شاملة لجميع السكان. ووفقاً للتعداد السكاني لعام 2015، كان 68% من السكان لديهم تأمين صحي، منهم 8.5% مشمولون بالتأمين من أكثر من جهة. والتأمين المُقدَّم من وزارة الصحة هو الأكثر انتشاراً، إذ يغطي 44.5% من السكان. ويغطي التأمين المُقدَّم من الخدمات الطبية الملكية 38% من السكان، ويحصل 17.5% من الأردنيين على تغطية تأمينية من خلال المستشفيات الجامعية والقطاع الخاص.[1]

ولكل مركز من المراكز الصحية منطقة مستهدفة مُحدَّدة بوضوح، فذلك شرط من شروط الاعتماد. ولكن نظراً إلى أن النظام الصحي في الأردن يتألف من قطاعات مختلفة غير مرتبطة بعضها ببعض، فغالباً ما يوجد ازدواج في السجلات الطبية، ويتعذر في بعض الأحيان تحديد المنطقة الخاصة بأحد مرافق الرعاية الصحية الأولية بسهولة.

وتوجد في جميع المرافق الصحية مبادئ توجيهية، ولكنها غير مُحدَّثة، كما أن بروتوكولات العلاج ليست في متناول جميع الموظفين. وهناك خُطط تدريبية مكتوبة مُدرجة في الخطط التشغيلية للمديريات، ولكن بعضها لا يُنفَّذ بسبب تحديات مالية. ويُطبَّق برنامج الاعتماد في الأردن على منشآت الرعاية الصحية الأولية التابعة لوزارة الصحة منذ عام 2010. وتستخدم جميع المراكز الصحية رقم تعريف شخصياً للسجلات الطبية. ولا يُطبَّق مبدأ تحديد طبيب أسرة أو ممارس عام واحد لكل أسرة.

وتشير الاستراتيجية الوطنية للقطاع الصحي في الأردن للأعوام 2016-2020 إلى طريقتين رئيسيتين لتحقيق التغطية الصحية الشاملة، ألا وهما: [1] حل طويل الأجل يتمثل في زيادة عدد الخريجين من أطباء الأسرة.[2، 3] [2] حل قصير الأجل يتمثل في تقليل العجز في عدد أطباء الأسرة من خلال تحسين قدرات الممارسين العامِّين في القطاع العام بأن يُقدَّم إليهم تدريب عبر الإنترنت.

التحديات الرئيسية التي تعترض تطبيق ممارسة طب الأسرة [4]

تشمل التحديات ما يلي: [1] محدودية وعي راسمي السياسات حول مفهوم ممارسة طب الأسرة، [2] سوء إدارة اللوجستيات وتوزيع المرافق الصحية والقوى العاملة، [3] الافتقار إلى شراكات بين القطاعين العام والخاص، [4] نقص الموارد والحوافز التي تضمن التطبيق السليم، [5] فشل برامج التدريب الحالية في تلبية الحاجة الهائلة إلى أطباء الأسرة، [6] محدودية الدعم القانوني والمالي المُقدَّم من أجل تطبيق ممارسة طب الأسرة.

سُبُل المضيّ قُدُماً

تشمل المبادرات ما يلي: [1] الحفاظ على الالتزام السياسي الرفيع المستوى، [2] إعادة هيكلة النظام الصحي لاستيعاب أطباء أسرة مُدرَّبين ومُعتمدين، [3] ضمان إطلاع الطلاب على طب الأسرة في المرحلة الجامعية، [4] ضمان تقديم دورات قصيرة لبناء قدرات الممارسين العامِّين في أثناء عملهم، [5] دعم المشاركة النشطة للقطاع الخاص، [6] التركيز على رضا العملاء ونظرة المجتمع إلى ممارسة طب الأسرة، [7] وضع خريطة طريق وطنية لتعزيز ممارسة طب الأسرة.

المراجع

1. الإصلاح الصحي الوطني، الأردن. 2018.
2. المكتب الإقليمي لمنظمة الصحة العالمية لشرق المتوسط، ل إ 63، 2016. توسيع نطاق طب الأسرة: التقدُّم المُحرز من أجل تحقيق التغطية الصحية الشاملة. EM/RC63/Tech.Disc.1. متاح على: http://www.emro.who.int/about-who/rc63/documentation.html.
3. المكتب الإقليمي لمنظمة الصحة العالمية لشرق المتوسط، ل إ 63، 2016. توسيع نطاق طب الأسرة: التقدُّم المُحرز من أجل تحقيق التغطية الصحية الشاملة. متاح على: http://applications.emro.who.int/docs/RC63_Resolutions_2016_R2_19197_EN.pdf?ua=1.
4. WHO EMRO. *Report on the Regional consultation on strengthening service provision through the family practice approach.* Cairo, Egypt, November 2014. WHO-EM/PHC/165/E. متاح على: http://apps.who.int/iris/bitstream/handle/10665/253400/IC_meet_rep_2015_EN_16267.pdf?sequence=1&isAllowed=y.

الكويت
هدى الدويسان، فاطمة أحمد بن ظفيري

103	العدد الإجمالي لمرافق الرعاية الصحية الأولية
832	عدد الممارسين العامّين العاملين في المرافق العامة للرعاية الصحية الأولية
194	عدد أطباء الأسرة المعتمدين العاملين في مرافق الرعاية الصحية الأولية
410	عدد أطباء الأسرة المعتمدين في مرافق الرعاية الصحية الأولية
35	متوسط عدد خريجي أطباء الأسرة كل سنة

مقدمة

في المناطق الصحية الست في الكويت، توفر مراكز الرعاية الصحية الأولية عيادات عامة، وعيادات للأمهات والأطفال، وعيادات لمرضى السكري، وعيادات الأسنان. كما تقدم المراكز خدمات الرعاية الوقائية والصحة المدرسية. وأُضيفت أيضاً في الآونة الأخيرة خدمات رعاية الصحة النفسية. وإضافةً إلى ذلك، أصبحت السجلات والبيانات الطبية مُحوسبة، ومن المقرر ربطها بشبكة المستشفيات الثانوية والتخصصية. ويبلغ حالياً العدد الإجمالي لمراكز الرعاية الصحية الأولية الخاضعة لإشراف وزارة الصحة 103 مراكز مُوزّعة على جميع المناطق. وبعض هذه المراكز يُطبق العناصر الثلاثة عشر لطب الأسرة، ويتفاوت تطبيقها في مراكز أخرى، مما يؤدي إلى وجود كلٍّ من مراكز صحة الأسرة والمراكز الصحية العامة. ويُقدِّم كل مركز خدماته الصحية لنحو 40 ألف نسمة من السكان. وتتمثل الخدمات المُقدَّمة في خدمات الممارسة العامة وطب الأسرة، وصحة

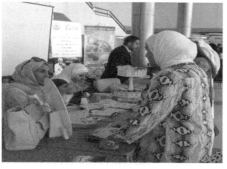

يوم مفتوح للمجتمع، مركز اليرموك

الأمهات، وصحة الأطفال، وخدمات طب الأسنان، والتطعيم، والخدمات الصحية الوقائية. وتوجد في المراكز أيضاً عيادات رعاية مرضى السكري، ومتابعة الأمراض المزمنة، وعيادات الصحة النفسية، ومختبرات، وصيدليات، ومرافق الأشعة السينية، وخدمات التمريض. وهناك أيضاً عيادات رعاية الرُضع وعيادات الإقلاع عن التدخين. وتوجد في جميع المراكز الصحية عيادات تستقبل المرضى دون مواعيد مسبقة، وشهدت الآونة الأخيرة التطبيق التجريبي لنظام عيادة عامة بالحجز المسبق في أحد مراكز صحة الأسرة.

واتسعت في الآونة الأخيرة قائمة الأدوية المتاحة في صيدليات مراكز الرعاية الصحية الأولية لتشمل أدوية جديدة. وتضم القائمة الآن أكثر من 200 دواء مختلف لأمراض الأطفال والبالغين والشيوخ. ويشمل التوسع أيضاً أدوية لأمراض مزمنة، مما يقلل من العبء المُلقى على عاتق المستشفيات المركزية.

وتستخدم مرافق الرعاية الصحية الأولية نظام الملفات الإلكترونية: "نظام معلومات الرعاية الأولية"، لتسجيل المعلومات الصحية للمرضى. ويشمل النظام عوامل الخطر الخاصة بالأمراض المزمنة غير السارية. ويشمل النظام حالياً جميع مراكز الرعاية الصحية الأولية. وسوف يجري قريباً ربط النظام بالمستشفيات. وتتَّبع مراكز الرعاية الصحية الأولية والأسرية بروتوكولات العلاج، وسياسات العمل، ومعايير الجودة عملاً بالمبادئ التوجيهية لمنظمة الصحة العالمية. وقد بدأ تطبيق بروتوكولات الجودة للحصول على الاعتماد الدولي، وذلك بالتعاون مع مجلس الاعتماد الكندي. وأُنشئ في عام 1983 برنامج الإقامة الطبية في طب الأسرة الذي تبلغ مدته 5 سنوات ويتبع الكلية الملكية للممارسين العامّين في المملكة المتحدة.

التحديات الرئيسية

إن معظم خدمات الرعاية الأولية في الكويت يُقدمها حالياً ممارسون عامُون يمثلون 64% من العدد الإجمالي للأطباء العاملين في الرعاية الأولية. ويمثل أطباء الأسرة المؤهلون النسبة المتبقية البالغة 36%. ويُعد تقليل أوقات انتظار المرضى أحد التحديات الرئيسية في تقديم الخدمات الصحية، وذلك بسبب ارتفاع أعداد المرضى واستنزاف طاقة أفراد الطاقم الطبي. وللتغلب على ذلك، تعتزم الحكومة بناء مزيد من المستشفيات ومراكز الرعاية الصحية الأولية، وتجديد وبناء مزيد من المختبرات الطبية، وتوسيع عيادات طب الأسنان، وذلك في إطار خطة التنمية الوطنية 2015 – 2019. [1] وتشمل التحديات الأخرى: [1] الحاجة إلى التقييم المنهجي لجودة الخدمات المُقدَّمة، [2] تحسين نظم الإحالة والمتابعة، [3] تنفيذ التدريب والتطوير المستمرين لموظفي تعزيز الصحة، [4] تعزيز الرعاية المنزلية والمجتمعية والنهوض بصحة المجتمع.

سُبُل المضيّ قُدُماً

تواصل دولة الكويت مساعيها الرامية إلى اتباع أفضل الممارسات لاستدامة الرعاية الصحية الأولية وممارسة طب الأسرة. ويعتمد التنفيذ الفعال لمبادرات جديدة على المناصرين لهذه المبادرات في مراكز الرعاية الصحية الأولية ووزارة الصحة. وقد ثبت في العقدين الماضيين أن التعاون مع شركاء دوليين ركيزةٌ رئيسيةٌ تسهم في تحقيق مستوى عالٍ من النجاح. وستواصل دولة الكويت بذل الجهود لاعتماد استراتيجيات وسياسات منظمة الصحة العالمية (WHO) والمنظمة العالمية لأطباء الأسرة (WONCA). وقد وضع المجلس الأعلى للتخطيط إطاراً للخطة الوطنية الخمسية لجميع الوزارات، ومنها وزارة الصحة.[2] وفيما يلي المجالات ذات الأولوية الاستراتيجية في الخدمات الصحية الوطنية ذات الصلة بالرعاية الصحية الأولية: [1] وضع نهج للرعاية الصحية الأولية يقوم على ممارسة طب الأسرة في جميع أنحاء البلد، [2] ضمان أن السجلات الصحية الإلكترونية قابلة للتشغيل المتبادل عبرواجهات الرعاية، [3] تنمية القدرات البحثية الخاصة بالخدمات الصحية للسماح بدورات مستمرة من التقييم والتحسين.

المراجع

1. *Kuwait National Development Plan 2035*. متاحة على: http://www.newkuwait.gov.kw/en/plan/ [22 أيلول/سبتمبر 2018].
2. *World Health Organization Report 2017*. *Development of a New National Health Sector Strategy for the State of Kuwait* (2018-2022).

تتوجه المؤلفتان بالشكر إلى السيدة هيفاء المضف على مساهمتها في جمع البيانات وتصميم هذا الفصل.

لبنان
وليد عمّار، أليسار راضي

العدد الإجمالي لمرافق الرعاية الصحية الأولية	205 مراكز للرعاية الصحية الأولية في الشبكة الوطنية الصحة العامة، من إجمالي 1100 مُستوصف*
عدد الممارسين العامِّين العاملين في المرافق العامة للرعاية الصحية الأولية**	غير متاح
عدد أطباء الأسرة المعتمدين العاملين في مرافق الرعاية الصحية الأولية	31 (في عام 2017)
متوسط عدد خريجي أطباء الأسرة كل سنة	10
عدد كليات الطب	6
عدد أقسام طب الأسرة	2

* أكثر من 95% من مراكز الرعاية الصحية الأولية تملكها وتديرها منظمات غير حكومية، فلا تملك أو تديروزارة الصحة العامة أو وزارة الشؤون الاجتماعية سوى عدد قليل جداً منها.

** عدد الممارسين العامِّين متذبذب بسبب ارتفاع معدل استبدال الموظفين.

مقدمة

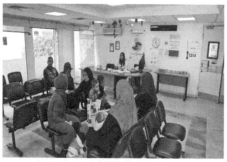
مرضى في أحد مراكز الرعاية الصحية الأولية

لقد اتسم النظام الصحي في لبنان على مدى العَقدين الماضيين بوجود شراكة طويلة الأمد بين القطاعين العام والخاص، ومجتمع مدني نشيط، وقطاع خاص مزدهر، وقطاع عام يستعيد بالتدريج دوره القيادي والتنظيمي. وتتكفل وزارة الصحة العامة بتكاليف الإقامة في المستشفيات والأدوية الباهظة الثمن للأشخاص غير المؤمَّن عليهم من خلال البرنامج المعني بالأمراض المستعصية. ويغطي الصندوق الوطني للضمان الاجتماعي وصناديق الموظفين الحكوميين نحو 40% من السكان، بينما يغطي التأمين الخاص نحو 8%. وتشتري وزارة الصحة العامة الخدمات الصحية من القطاعين الخاص والعام من أجل السكان غير المشمولين بالتأمين الصحي الذين تبلغ نسبتهم 52%. وتشتري الوزارة الخدمات الصحية من المستشفيات الخاصة، بنظام الحصص وبأسعار موحدة، من خلال اتفاقيات تعاقدية. وتقدم الوزارة دعماً مالياً جزئياً إلى المستشفيات العامة، وتشتري منها الخدمات أيضاً. كما تدعم الوزارة خدمات الرعاية الصحية الأولية، من خلال المساهمة العينية بالأدوية واللقاحات والتدريبات.[1]

وعلى مدى العقود الثلاثة الماضية، وضعت الوزارة خيارات للإصلاحات الخاصة بدفع ثمن الخدمة إلى مُقدمي الرعاية في العيادات الخارجية، وشرعت في تطبيق نظام اعتماد بشأن الرعاية الصحية الأولية بما في ذلك مبادئ توجيهية لوضع المعايير، وكذلك متطلبات المرافق المادية والقُوى العاملة والمعدات والنظم التشغيلية. كما أنشأت الوزارة شبكة وطنية لمراكز الرعاية الصحية الأولية، واتسعت هذه الشبكة تدريجياً على مر السنين لتشمل معظم المناطق الجغرافية في البلد، مع زيادة التركيز على مناطق الفئات السكانية الضعيفة. وتوفر الشبكة الوطنية لمراكز الرعاية الصحية الأولية أدوية أساسية وخدمات صحية أساسية، مثل طب الأطفال، وطب الأسرة، وصحة الفم، والصحة الإنجابية، وطب القلب، والتطعيم. وشرعت الوزارة في العمل على وضع آلية اعتماد لمؤسسات الرعاية الصحية الأولية، من أجل مراقبة الجودة وضمانها.[2]

التحديات الرئيسية

[1] النهوض بطب الأسرة: يُعد تحفيز الممارسين العامّين على تلقي تدريب نظاميّ في مجال طب الأسرة إحدى العقبات الرئيسية التي تعوق اتباع نهج طب الأسرة الذي يركز على الناس. ولا يوجد في لبنان لوائح تحدّ من عدد الاختصاصيين، أو تحدد توزيع الأطباء على التخصصات والمناطق الجغرافية. [2] تكييف تقديم الخدمات الصحية حسب نهج ممارسة طب الأسرة في مراكز الرعاية الصحية الأولية: النموذج الحالي لتقديم الخدمات من خلال شبكة مراكز الرعاية الصحية الأولية التابعة لوزارة الصحة العامة لا يتلاءم تلاؤماً تاماً مع دور طبيب الأسرة على النحو المُبيّن في النهج الذي يركز على الناس. ولطبيب الأسرة سلطة محدودة في اتخاذ القرارات الخاصة بتنظيم الرعاية الصحية.[3] [3] تغيير ثقافة الرعاية المتخصصة: الوصول إلى الرعاية المتخصصة متاح بسهولة، والنهوض بالرعاية الأساسية الشاملة عن طريق ممارسة طب الأسرة يتطلب جهداً. ويحتاج ذلك إلى خدمات مدفوعة الثمن مقدماً ولوائح بشأن الأطراف الأخرى التي تدفع. [4] الحصول على تأييد أصحاب المصلحة من أجل إدماج أطباء الأسرة: عند اعتماد نهج طب الأسرة، سينخفض عدد الحالات في العيادات الخاصة وسينخفض دخل الاختصاصيين. ولذلك فإن تفادي معارضتهم لنهج طب الأسرة يمثل تحدياً مهماً.

سُبُل المضيّ قُدُماً

رغم التحديات والقيود، يوجد عزم قوي على المضي قدماً نحو تعزيز الرعاية الصحية الأولية. ويتطلب ذلك نقلة نوعية لأطباء الأسرة ليكونوا في قلب نظام رعاية صحية أولية يركز على الناس. وتوجد فرصة كبيرة ليشارك بنشاط مزيد من أصحاب المصلحة في هذه النقلة. وفيما يلي التوصيات الرئيسية: [1] فتح الباب أمام مراكز الممارسة الخاصة/عيادات أطباء الأسرة للمساهمة في جهود الرعاية الأولية وتشجيع وزارة الصحة العامة على تجربة خطط السداد على أساس الفرد، [2] السعي إلى توفير الرعاية الصحية الأولية من خلال نهج أشمل، مثل تطوير مفاهيم المدن الصحية/القرى الصحية، [3] إعادة طبيب الأسرة إلى وضعه الطبيعي في صميم آلية إحالة داخل الرعاية الصحية الأولية، [4] الإشراف على نظام إحالة واضح، ومراقبة التدخلات المجتمعية المنحى.

المراجع

1. وزارة الصحة العامة. الخطة الاستراتيجية للمدة المتوسطة (2016 إلى 2020). لبنان؛ 2016. متاحة على: https://www.moph.gov.lb/userfiles/files/%D9%90Announcement/Final-StrategicPlanHealth2017.pdf [جرى الاطلاع عليها في 19 نيسان/أبريل 2018].
2. Ministry of Public Health. Accreditation of primary health care centers and quality of care; 2016.
3. Helou, M, Rizk, GA. State of family medicine practice in Lebanon. **Journal of Family Medicine and Primary Care,** 2016;5(1):51–5. متاح على: https://www.ncbi.nlm.nih.gov/pubmed/27453843 [جرى الاطلاع عليه في 22 أيلول/سبتمبر 2018].

ليبيا

سيد جعفر حسين

1355، منها 273 مرفقاً مغلقاً بسبب النزاع	العدد الإجمالي لمرافق الرعاية الصحية الأولية
2135	عدد الممارسين العامّين العاملين في المرافق العامة للرعاية الصحية الأولية
30	عدد أطباء الأسرة المعتمدين العاملين في مرافق الرعاية الصحية الأولية
10	متوسط عدد خريجي أطباء الأسرة كل سنة
14	عدد كليات الطب
10	عدد أقسام طب الأسرة

مقدمة

أعاق النزاع المسلح تقديم معظم الخدمات الصحية الأساسية التي يحتاج إليها الليبيون، لا سيما الفئات الضعيفة. فقد أُغلِق كثير من المراكز الطبية والمستشفيات الخاصة في المناطق المتضررة من النزاع بسبب عدم وجود ما يكفي من الإمدادات أو الأيدي العاملة أو الكهرباء، مما يجعل من الصعب حصول المواطنين على الرعاية الصحية التي يحتاجون إليها. ويشير التقدير الذي أجري مؤخراً إلى إغلاق 17 مستشفى و273 مرفقاً من مرافق الرعاية الصحية الأولية.[1] وتُقدَّم خدمات الرعاية الصحية الأولية من خلال شبكة واسعة تتألف من 1355 مرفقاً من مرافق الرعاية الصحية الأولية (بما في ذلك وحدات الرعاية الصحية، ومراكز الرعاية الصحية، والعيادات الشاملة). وأُغلِق 20% من هذه المرافق في عام 2017.[1] ويرى كثير من

مركز رعاية صحية أولية بمدينة تاجوراء

الليبيين أن خدمات الرعاية الصحية الأولية لا تكاد تقدم شيئاً إلى المرضى، ولذلك يميل الناس إلى تخطي مستوى الرعاية الصحية الأولية بسبب انخفاض مستوى جودة الخدمات، ويتوجهون مباشرةً إلى العيادات الخارجية أو أقسام الطوارئ في مستشفيات الرعاية الثانوية أو التخصصية. ولا يوجد في كثير من مراكز الرعاية الصحية الأولية أطباء متفرغون، وإن وُجِدوا فإنهم عادةً ما يكونون حديثي العهد بالعمل ولا يتمتعون بخبرة كبيرة.

ويختلف مستوى المراكز والوحدات الصحية العاملة في الشعبيات اختلافاً كبيراً عنه في طرابلس التي بها أكبر عدد من المرافق العاملة. ويشير تحليل متعمق إلى أن 70% من الأدوية المُدرجة في قائمة الأدوية الأساسية غير متوفرة، ولذلك يحثُّ الأطباءُ المرضى على شراء الأدوية من القطاع الخاص أو البحث عنها في المراكز الأخرى أو العيادات الشاملة أو المستشفيات. ويمتلك الموظفون قدرات ضعيفة، إذ لم يتلقَّ أحد منهم تدريباً في مجال طب الأسرة، ولا يخضعون للرقابة، ولا يشاركون في أي تطوير مهني مستمر. ولا توجد لدى معظم المرافق سجلات طبية إلكترونية أو ورقية تُدوَّن فيها معلومات أساسية عن سكان المناطق الخاصة بالمرافق. وتفتقر مرافق الرعاية الصحية الأولية إلى التصميم الموحد، وليس لديها قائمة بالمعدات الأساسية والمختبرات التي تُمكِّن المرفق من تقديم رعاية عالية الجودة. ويعتقد كثيرون أن اللجوء إلى الرعاية الصحية الأولية في أي مشكلة صحية خطيرة سيُسفر عن إحالة المريض إلى طبيب متخصص، ولذلك فإنهم يتخطون الرعاية الصحية الأولية اختصاراً للوقت.

التحديات الرئيسية

تواجه المحاولات التي تُبذَل لتحديث تقديم الخدمات الصحية عوائق أمنية وسياسية ومالية خطيرة، فضلاً عن العوائق الخطيرة المتعلقة بالقوى العاملة و"مقاومة التغيير". وتواجه الخدمات الصحية في الوقت الحالي تحديات جسيمة. فالنظام

الصحي يتسم بالضعف، وأداؤه العام ينطوي على أوجه قصور، بما في ذلك:[2] [1] عدم وجود سياسة صحية تقنية ومهام تخطيطية داخل إدارة التخطيط، [2] الضعف العام في القدرة المؤسسية على التخطيط للبرامج الصحية وتنفيذها على المستويين الوطني ودون الوطني، [3] عدم كفاية نُظُم المعلومات الصحية الوطنية وتفككها في مجالات البيانات اللازمة لاتخاذ القرارات، والبنية التحتية لتكنولوجيا المعلومات والاتصالات، وتطوير السجلات الإلكترونية لقطاع الصحة، [4] عدم وجود سياسة بشأن تمويل الرعاية الصحية، وعدم وجود خيارات لمخططات التغطية الشاملة، [5] عدم وجود خطة وسياسية واستراتيجية وطنية واضحة لتنمية الموارد البشرية، والافتقار إلى نظام شامل للتطوير المهني المستمر.

وتشمل التحديات الرئيسية لممارسة طب الأسرة ما يلي: [1] قلة عدد أطباء الأسرة الذين يتخرجون كل عام، [2] عدم وجود صندوق مُخصَّص لتقديم خدمات ممارسة طب الأسرة، [3] عدم وجود مسار وظيفي مهني معتمَد لأطباء الأسرة، [4] النظر إلى أطباء الأسرة على أنهم تهديد لتخصصات أخرى، [5] انعدام التنسيق بين وزارة الصحة ووزارة التعليم، [6] انخفاض مستوى إقبال المجتمع على أطباء الأسرة، [7] عدم إدراج ممارسة طب الأسرة ضمن الأولويات العليا لوزارة الصحة خلال الأزمة الحالية.

سُبُل المضيّ قُدُماً

اتَّبعت ليبيا نهج تحسين الرعاية الصحية الأولية من خلال التعزيز التدريجي لنموذج صحة الأسرة. وهناك التزام سياسي بتوسيع نطاق طب الأسرة على الرغم من التحديات الهائلة وتصدُّع النظام الصحي، وذلك ببعض المخصصات المالية للبرنامج الوطني. ويتبنى نموذج صحة الأسرة خطة إصلاحية شاملة بحيث: [1] تكون وزارة الصحة مسؤولة عن جميع خدمات الرعاية الأولية، وتُقدَّم هذه الخدمات مجاناً لجميع العاملين والمقيمين في ليبيا، [2] لا تمنح الحكومة ترخيصاً لأي جهة تُقدِّم خدمات الرعاية الأولية ولا تكون جزءاً من خدمات وزارة الصحة (من خلال الخدمة المباشرة أو التعاقدية) لضمان الإنصاف والحفاظ على جودة الخدمة وكمالها وشموليتها، [3] تستكشف وزارة الصحة الحوافز اللازمة لجذب مهنيين صحيين ذوي كفاءة عالية إلى العمل في مجال الرعاية الصحية الأولية، بما في ذلك تدريبهم على طب الأسرة.

المراجع

1. World Health Organization. The Service Availability and Readiness Assessment survey in Libya. 2017 (SARA). متاح على: http://www.who.int/hac/crises/lby/en/ [جرى الاطلاع عليه في 20 نيسان/أبريل 2018].

2. 2017 Review of Health Sector in Libya. https://reliefweb.int/report/Libya/2017-review-health-sector-libya

المغرب
أمينة ساهل، حفيظ هشري

العدد الإجمالي لمرافق الرعاية الصحية الأولية	2759 (760 منها يديرها ممرضون في مناطق ريفية[1])
عدد الممارسين العامّين العاملين في المرافق العامة للرعاية الصحية الأولية	3100
عدد أطباء الأسرة المعتمدين العاملين في مرافق الرعاية الصحية الأولية	45
متوسط عدد خريجي أطباء الأسرة كل سنة	40

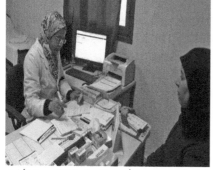

طبيبة مع مريضة في أحد مرافق الرعاية الصحية الأولية

مقدمة

بعد التوقيع على إعلان ألما-آتا، وضع المغرب الاستراتيجية الخاصة بالرعاية الصحية الأولية ضمن أولويات الحكومة في العمل من أجل الصحة. وكانت أول خطة خمسية للمغرب بشأن الرعاية الصحية الأولية تشمل الفترة من 1981 إلى 1985. وبدأ بدعم من شركاء تقنيين وماليين تنفيذ العديد من المشاريع القطاعية التي تستهدف تطوير الرعاية الصحية الأولية. وقدمت هذه المشاريع مساهمات كبيرة في تحسين التغطية الصحية وتوحيد نهج التغطية وإعادة هيكلة البرامج الصحية.

وحدث تحسن كبير في التغطية التي أتاحتها مرافق الرعاية الصحية الأولية للسكان. وزاد عدد مرافق الرعاية الصحية الأولية من 1653 مرفقاً في عام 1990 إلى 2689 مرفقاً في عام 2014، [1] وإلى 2759 مرفقاً في عام 2015، بزيادة قدرها 72% على مدار 25 عاماً[2]. وتحسنت الخدمة بوجه عام بنسبة 19%، مع زيادة نسبة المرافق إلى السكان من 1:14600 في عام 1990 إلى 1:11600 في عام 2015 (بأرقام تتراوح من 1:4400 كحد أقصى إلى 1:19750 كحد أدنى). وتغيرت نسبة أفراد التمريض إلى السكان تغيراً طفيفاً بين عامي 2007 و2011 (من 1:3267 في عام 2009 إلى 1:3327 في عام 2011)، بينما انخفضت التغطية التي يقدمها الممارسون العامُون في القطاع العام في مرافق الرعاية الصحية الأولية من 1.01:10000 إلى 0.94:10000 نسمة، بل كانت التغطية أقل من ذلك في المناطق الريفية .

وعلى الرغم من الجهود التي بذلتها وزارة الصحة في بناء مرافق الرعاية الصحية الأولية، فإن النسبة المئوية للسكان الذين يعيشون على مسافة تزيد على ستة كيلومترات من أي مرفق من هذه المرافق ظلت مرتفعة، إذ بلغت 43%، ولا تزال التغطية المتنقلة بديلاً قيّماً.

كما أن حزمة الخدمات الصحية المُقدَّمة تُحدَّد على المستوى الوطني وحسب نوع مرفق الرعاية الصحية الأولية. وأُعيد تشكيل حزمة الخدمات الصحية في ضوء التحول الوبائي والسكاني الجاري في المغرب.[3] وتشمل حزمة الخدمات الصحية الحالية تغطية الأمراض المزمنة، لا سيما أمراض القلب والأوعية الدموية ومرض السكري، فضلاً عن تحري الإصابة بسرطان الثدي وسرطان عنق الرحم. وجرى في الآونة الأخيرة استعراض حزمة الخدمات الصحية وإعادة تحديدها في إطار مشروع لتعزيز نظام الرعاية الصحية. وباستثناء حالات الطوارئ، يكون الانتقال من مستوى إلى آخر من خلال نظام الإحالة. كما أن نظام المعلومات مُجزّأ، ومُوجّه نحو برامج صحية رأسية، ولا يُركّز على المرضى وأسرهم. وقدمت وزارة الصحة طائفة متنوعة من مقاييس الجودة لغرس ثقافة الجودة في مرافق الرعاية الصحية الأولية.

التحديات الرئيسية لتنفيذ ممارسة طب الأسرة

تشمل التحديات ما يلي: [1] ضعْف الالتزام السياسي، نظراً إلى أن الدراسات الطبية لم تشهد، حتى الآن، أي تعديل لإدخال تخصص طب الأسرة في كليات الطب المغربية. وعلاوة على ذلك، لم تعلن وزارة الصحة رسمياً عن إصلاحها للرعاية الصحية الأولية بناء على ممارسة طب الأسرة. [2] افتقار أطباء الأسرة إلى التدريب. [3] عدم كفاية اللوائح التنظيمية والدعم المالي لتطبيق ممارسة طب الأسرة. [4] عدم تسجيل السكان لدى أطباء الرعاية الصحية الأولية. [5] قصور نظام التوجيه والافتقار إلى آليات استقاء الآراء. [6] ضعف التزام القطاع الخاص ومشاركته. [7] عدم رضا المجتمع عن خدمات الرعاية الصحية الأولية العامة.

سُبُل المضيّ قُدُماً

يتجسد التزام وزارة الصحة السياسي بتعزيز ممارسة طب الأسرة في الاستراتيجية الصحية الوطنية للفترة من 2012 إلى 2016 وفي خطة العمل القطاعية الجديدة للفترة من 2019 إلى 2025 التي تدعو إلى تطوير الرعاية الصحية الأولية وتصحيح دور الممارسين العامّين في تنفيذ برنامج الدولة التدريبي الخاص بصحة الأسرة والمجتمع. وينبغي تعزيز هذا الالتزام السياسي من خلال التزام أصحاب المصلحة الآخرين المشاركين في تطوير ممارسة طب الأسرة، مثل كليات الطب ونقابة الأطباء ووزارة المالية. وقد أصدرت وزارة الصحة مشروع مرسوم بشأن إقامة شراكات مع الممارسين العامّين والاختصاصيين والصيادلة وجرّاحي الأسنان في القطاع الخاص، ويسمح هذا المرسوم بإبرام اتفاقيات تعاقدية للعمل بدوام جزئي في المرافق الصحية العامة، حسب توفرها وحسب المهارات المطلوبة في كل منطقة صحية. واتسع نطاق هذه الشراكة بين القطاعين العام والخاص بإشراك القطاع الخاص في الاستراتيجيات والبرامج الرامية إلى معالجة مجموعة من القضايا الصحية ذات الأولوية.

المراجع

1. وزارة الصحة، المغرب. الاستراتيجية القطاعية للصحة 2012–2016. متاحة على: https://www.mind-bank.info/item/3714 [جرى الاطلاع عليها في 22 أيلول/سبتمبر 2018].

2. Ministry of Health, Morocco. Hospitals and Ambulatory Health Department Database. 2017.

3. Ministry of Health, Morocco. Health Coverage by the Basic Health Care Network. Methodological Guide for the Production of an Extension Plan. 1990.

عُمان

سعيد اللمكي، أحمد سالم سيف المنظري

235	العدد الإجمالي لمرافق الرعاية الصحية الأولية
3837	عدد الممارسين العامِّين العاملين في المرافق العامة للرعاية الصحية الأولية
143	عدد أطباء الأسرة المعتمدين العاملين في مرافق الرعاية الصحية الأولية
20–16	متوسط عدد خريجي أطباء الأسرة كل سنة
2	عدد كليات الطب
2	عدد أقسام طب الأسرة

مقدمة

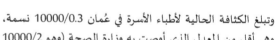

يستند نظام تقديم خدمات الرعاية الأولية إلى أسس راسخة، ويقوم على مبادئ واضحة. ويعتمد حجم هياكل مرافق الرعاية الصحية الأولية ونوع هذه الهياكل على عدد السكان، والمسافة بينها وبين المستشفيات/مراكز الإحالة الأخرى، والخدمات اللوجستية.[1]

وتُصنَّف مرافق الرعاية الصحية الأولية عموماً إلى مراكز صحية، ومجمعات صحية (بها عيادة ولادة)، وعيادات شاملة، ومستشفيات محلية.

ويعمل في مرافق الرعاية الصحية الأولية ممارسون عامُّون، وممرضون، وصيادلة، وصيادلة مساعدون، وأطباء أسنان، وممرضون مساعدون لأطباء الأسنان، وتقنيو مختبرات، واختصاصيو تصوير شُعاعيّ، ومُثقِّفون صحيون، واختصاصيو تغذية، ومضمِّدون، وموظفو سجلات طبية، وسائقون.

وتبلغ الكثافة الحالية لأطباء الأسرة في عُمان 10000/0.3 نسمة، وهي أقل من المعدل الذي أوصت به وزارة الصحة (وهو 10000/2

صحة المجتمع – زيارة منزلية

نسمة، بناء على توصيات قرار وزراء مجلس التعاون الخليجي، الكويت 2007).[2] وتقل كثافة الممرضين عن المعيار الأوروبي البالغ 100000/65 نسمة.[3]

وتُعتبر المراكز الصحية الجهة الأولى التي يلجأ إليها جميع المواطنين والمقيمين للحصول على الخدمات الصحية. وهذه المراكز تدعمها مستشفيات الإحالة على المستوى المحلي والإقليمي وعلى مستوى الولايات (المحافظات).

ويُحال المرضى من مركز أو مرفق الرعاية الصحية الأولية إلى مستوى رعاية أعلى به خدمات أكثر تطوراً، مثل خدمات المرضى الداخليين أو الجراحة أو العناية المركزة.

ويُحال المرضى، بوجه عام، من مركز صحي إلى المستشفى المحلي أو إلى العيادة الشاملة. وقد وُضِع دليل شامل لتنظيم وتوجيه عملية الإحالة والإحالة المرتدة (2004). ولم يُحدَّث بعض الأدلة منذ ذلك الحين.

التحديات الرئيسية

على الرغم من الإنجازات المذكورة أعلاه، تواجه الرعاية الصحية الأولية عدة تحديات، نذكر منها أن: [1] معظم مرافق الرعاية الصحية الأولية مساحتها صغيرة جداً، وغرف الاستشارة بها غير كافية، وتكاد تخلو من الأماكن والمعدات المخصصة لاستقبال الحالات الطارئة، [2] خدمات الدعم غير كافية، بما في ذلك المختبر وخدمات التصوير الشُّعاعي وخدمات التشخيص والأجهزة، [3] هناك نقصاً في موظفي الرعاية الصحية المهرة مثل أطباء الأسرة، [4] حجم الأمراض المزمنة في تزايد، [5] هناك تهديدات ناشئة حديثاً للصحة العامة العالمية .

سُبُل المضيّ قُدُماً

تسببت الأمراض السارية في الماضي في حدوث زيادة كبيرة في معدل المراضة والوفيات بعُمان، ولكن بدأت تظهر في السنوات الأخيرة أنماط جديدة من المراضة بسبب أمراض غير سارية أو مرتبطة بأسلوب المعيشة وبسبب التغير المستمر لهيكل توزيع أعمار السكان. وقد أظهرت نتائج المسح الصحي الوطني لعام 2000، الذي أجرته وزارة الصحة، صورة مقلقة لعوامل الخطر الخاصة بالأمراض غير السارية. وتشير إحصائيات المراضة في عام 2011 الخاصة بالمرافق الصحية التابعة لوزارة الصحة أن الأمراض غير السارية وراء نحو 49.9% من جميع زيارات المرضى الخارجيين، و37.6% من حالات دخول المستشفيات.[3] وقد أدى ذلك إلى حدوث تحوُّل مهم في برامج الرعاية الصحية الأولية، إذ توجَّه التركيز نحو الأمراض غير السارية وخدمات الرعاية الصحية الأولية مثل: [1] **العيادات الصغيرة لمرضى السكري**: حيث لا يكاد يخلو مركز صحي من عيادة صغيرة لمرضى السكري. وتتوفر هذه الخدمة الأدوية الأساسية لعلاج السكري.[4] [2] **خدمات رعاية القدم السكرية**: منذ عام 2008 يُقدَّم تثقيف صحي منظَّم بشأن رعاية القدم السكرية، بالإضافة إلى مبادئ توجيهية لتقييم القدم السكرية وعلاجها.[5] [3] **خدمات مرضى ضغط الدم المرتفع**: تلقَّى الأطباء والممرضون العاملون في مواقع الرعاية الصحية الأولية تدريباً على تشخيص ارتفاع ضغط الدم وعلاج المرضى المصابين به. [4] **خدمات الأمراض النفسية**: يُعد دمج خدمات الصحة النفسية في الرعاية الأولية أصلح وسيلة لضمان حصول الأشخاص على الرعاية الصحية النفسية التي يحتاجون إليها. [5] **برنامج التحري عن الأمراض غير السارية**: يهدف هذا البرنامج إلى فحص مَنْ تزيد أعمارهم عن 40 عاماً من أجل الكشف المبكر عن الأمراض غير السارية والوقاية منها، لا سيما ارتفاع ضغط الدم والسكري وفرط شَحْميَّات الدم والبدانة وأمراض الكلى. [6] **رعاية المسنين**: توفر رعاية المسنين تقييماً شاملاً للمرضى المسنين وتدخلات مناسبة مثل التدخل السريري والعلاج الطبيعي الذي تقدمه وحدات العلاج الطبيعي المتنقلة، وتدخلات اجتماعية، وخدمات إحالة.

المراجع

1. وثائق النظرة المستقبلية للرعاية الصحية الأولية لعام 2050 التي عُرضت في مؤتمر النظرة المستقبلية للرعاية الصحية عُمان 2050. أيار/مايو 2012.

2. وزارة الصحة، سلطنة عمان. الخطة الخمسية الثامنة للتنمية الصحية، 2011- 2015. متاحة على: http://www.nationalplanningcycles.org/sites/default/files/country_docs/Oman/five_year_plan_for_health_development_2011-2015.pdf [جرى الاطلاع عليها في 17 نيسان/أبريل 2018].

3. وزارة الصحة، سلطنة عمان. 2016. التقرير الصحي السنوي 2016.

4. International Diabetes Federation IDF Diabetes Atlas (Eighth edition). 2017 متاح على: http://www.diabetesatlas.org/ [جرى الاطلاع عليه في 17 نيسان/أبريل 2018].

5. Al-Lawati, JA, Al-Riyami, AM, Mohammed, AJ, Jousilahti, P. Increasing prevalence of diabetes mellitus in Oman. *Diabetic Medicine. . 2002, 19 (11): 954–957.* متاح على: https://onlinelibrary.wiley.com/doi/pdf/10.1046/j.1464-5491.2002.00818.x [17 نيسان/أبريل 2018].

باكستان
واريس كيداوي، ماري أندراديس، ضياء الحق، كشميرا نانجي

العدد الإجمالي لمرافق الرعاية الصحية الأولية	11530
عدد الممارسين العامّين العاملين في المرافق العامة للرعاية الصحية الأولية	البيانات غير متوفرة
عدد أطباء الأسرة المعتمدين العاملين في مرافق الرعاية الصحية الأولية	18
متوسط عدد خريجي أطباء الأسرة كل سنة	البيانات غير متوفرة
عدد كليات الطب*	107
عدد أقسام طب الأسرة	7

*41 كلية حكومية و66 كلية خاصة

مقدمة

تتسم خدمات الرعاية الصحية الأولية بأنها خدمات مجتمعية قائمة على المرافق. ومن العاملين في مجال صحة المجتمع: العاملات الصحيات، والقابلات المجتمعيات، والقائمون على التطعيم، والمفتشون الصحيون.[1] وتوجد نحو 92900 عاملة صحية (0.43 عاملة لكل 1000 نسمة) يُقدمن خدمات الرعاية الصحية الأولية على مستوى المجتمعات المحلية. وتُقدَّم الخدمات القائمة على المرافق من خلال شبكة من المستوصفات المدنية، والوحدات الصحية الأساسية، والمراكز الصحية الريفية.[2] وقد تختلف الجوانب الزمنية لتقديم الخدمات من مرفق إلى آخر.

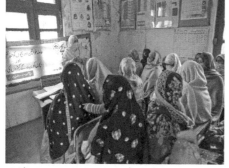
متابعة ما بعد الولادة في أحد مرافق الرعاية الصحية الأولية

وفي سبيل تحقيق الرعاية الصحية الشاملة، أطلقت الحكومة الاتحادية وحكومات الأقاليم مبادرات اجتماعية لحماية الصحة من أجل توفير الحماية المالية لسكانها. وتشير التقديرات إلى أن القطاع الخاص يقدم ما يتراوح بين 70% و80% من خدمات العيادات الخارجية.[3] وتُبذل محاولات لتقديم خدمات تنظيم الأسرة على مستوى مرافق الرعاية الصحية الأولية وعلى مستوى المجتمعات المحلية، بما في ذلك تقديم المشورة بشأن المباعدة بين الولادات، واستخدام تكنولوجيات حديثة، وتمكين المرأة من تنظيم الأسرة. وتتمثل المكونات الأساسية لخدمات الرعاية الصحية الأولية في التحصين الروتيني، والتأهب لطوارئ وكوارث الصحة العامة، والإعاقة، والصحة النفسية، وصحة الفم. وأجريت دراسات محدودة لتقييم مدى الرضا عن جودة الخدمات المُقدَّمة من مركز الرعاية الصحية الأولية. وتشير الأدبيّات المتاحة إلى أن مستوى رضا المرضى عن المستشفيات الخاصة أكبر من مستوى رضاهم عن القطاع العام. وتصل معدلات عدم الرضا عن القطاع العام إلى 80%.

التحديات الرئيسية

يبلغ العدد الإجمالي لمرافق الرعاية الصحية الأولية 11530 مرفقاً، ويتولى إدارةَ هذه المرافق ممارسون عامُّون. ولكن هناك 18 مرفقاً فقط يديرها أطباء أسرة معتمَدون. ولا يوجد في كليات الطب البالغ عددها 107 كليات سوى أربعة أقسام لطبّ الأسرة. ويختلف توفر حزمة الخدمات الصحية الأساسية من مقاطعة إلى أخرى حسب موقعها. ولا يوجد حالياً نظام جيد لممارسة طب الأسرة. ولا ينصبُّ التركيز في المقام الأول على الوقاية، مما يؤدي إلى عدم إدماج طب الأسرة في النظام الصحي. ولم تُدرَج الأمراض غير السارية ورعاية المسنين ومشاكل الصحة النفسية في حزمة الخدمات الصحية. ولا بد من تعزيز نظام المعلومات

الصحية والترصد لأن معظم المعلومات الواردة غيردقيقة ولا يُستفاد منها شيء. ومن التحديات الأخرى أن الأطباء الاختصاصيين يتوهمون أن تطبيق نموذج الرعاية الصحية الأسرية في الخطوط الأمامية يمثل تهديداً لعملهم. وقد بُذلت محاولات لإقامة شراكات بين القطاعين العام والخاص كنموذج جديد للخدمات الصحية في مجال ممارسة طب الأسرة، إلا أن هذه الشراكات لم تحقق نجاحاً كبيراً بسبب عدم وضوح آلية التعاقد مع القطاع الخاص، وعدم وجود مؤشرات مُحدَّدة بوضوح لقياس الأداء والنتائج. ويوجد أكثر من 168000 طبيب مُسجَّل، وحتى على افتراض أن نصفهم من الممارسين العامِّين، فإنه عدد هائل، ولا بد أن يتلقوا تدريباً لتعزيز كفاءاتهم كأطباء أسرة.

سُبُل المضيّ قُدُماً

يمكن أن تؤدي ممارسة طب الأسرة دوراً حاسماً في تحسين المؤشرات الصحية لأي بلد. ولم يسبق للحكومة أن أبدت رغبتها في جعل ممارسة طب الأسرة جزءاً لا يتجزّأ من النظام الصحي. فقد حدَّدت الرؤية الصحية الوطنية للفترة 2016-2020 ثمانية أركان مواضيعية للنظام الصحي، ألا وهي: التمويل الصحي، وتقديم الخدمات الصحية، والموارد البشرية، ونُظُم المعلومات الصحية، والحوكمة، والأدوية والتكنولوجيات الأساسية، والصلات الشاملة لعدة قطاعات، والمسؤوليات الصحية العالمية.

ولكي تنجح ممارسة طب الأسرة من حيث القدرة على تحمُّل التكاليف، والإتاحة، وجودة الرعاية، يجب أن يحدث تواصل مع المجتمع من خلال خدمات الرعاية الصحية المنزلية، وأن توجد علاقة قوية بمراكز الرعاية الثانوية والتخصصية. ولا بد من ربط مراكز ممارسة طب الأسرة بالمنظمات غير الحكومية الأخرى التي تعمل بالفعل في هذا المجال، من أجل سد الثغرات الموجودة في الخدمات عند الاقتضاء. فإقامة روابط مع دُور التوليد الخاصة الجيدة ستساعد على توفير الرعاية التوليدية. وإضافةً إلى ذلك، يلزم ربط خطط التأمين الصحي الحكومية بممارسة طب الأسرة من أجل إتاحة الخدمات للسكان بتكلفة ميسورة.

المراجع

1. Sixth Five-Year Plan 1978–1983, Chapter 19: Towards a Comprehensive National Coverage. Planning Commission, Government of Pakistan. متاح على: http://www.pakistan.gov.pk/ministries/planninganddevelopment-ministry/index.htm [كانون الأول/ديسمبر 2017].

2. Hafeez A, Mohamud BK, Shiekh MR, Shah SAI, Jooma R. Lady health workers programme in Pakistan: challenges, achievements and the way forward. *JPMA*, 2011; 61(3): 210.

3. Malik MA, Gul W, Iqbal SP, Abrejo F. Cost of primary health care in Pakistan. *Journal of Ayub Medical College Abbottabad, 2015; 27(1): 88–92.*

فلسطين

رند سلمان، جيرالد أوكنشاوب، أسعد الرملاوي

المجموع	قطاع غزة	الضفة الغربية	المؤشر
		الإقليم	
739	152	587	مرافق الرعاية الصحية الأولية (وزارة الصحة والأونروا والمنظمات غير الحكومية والدوائر العسكرية)
6416	1745	4671	الممارسون العامُون
553	153	400	الممارسون العامُون العاملون في المرافق العامة للرعاية الصحية الأولية التابعة لوزارة الصحة
61	21 في مرافق وزارة الصحة، و15 في الأونروا	25 داخل مرافق وزارة الصحة	أطباء الأسرة المعتمدون العاملون في مرافق الرعاية الصحية الأولية
	غير مُبلغ عنه	5-3 كل سنة	متوسط عدد خريجي أطباء الأسرة كل سنة
4	2 (في الجامعة الإسلامية وفرع جامعة القدس)	2 (في جامعتي النجاح والقدس)	كليات الطب
2	1 (جامعة الأزهر)	1 (جامعة النجاح)	أقسام طب الأسرة
6	3	3	مراكز التدريب على طب الأسرة بوزارة الصحة

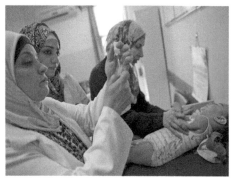

تطعيم في أحد مرافق الرعاية الصحية الأولية

مقدمة

تتولى تقديمَ خدمات الرعاية الصحية الأولية في فلسطين وزارةُ الصحة، ومنظمات غير حكومية، ووكالة الأمم المتحدة لإغاثة وتشغيل اللاجئين (الأونروا)، ودوائر طبية عسكرية، والقطاع الخاص.1 ويوجد 4671 ممارساً عاماً يعملون في الضفة الغربية و1745 ممارساً عاماً يعملون في قطاع غزة. ويعمل 400 ممارس عام في عيادات الرعاية الصحية الأولية التابعة لوزارة الصحة في الضفة الغربية، و153 ممارساً عاماً في عيادات وزارة الصحة في غزة. ويعاني نظام الرعاية الصحية الأولية في فلسطين نقصاً عاماً في الموظفين بالإضافة إلى عجز في عدد أطباء الأسرة المُدرَّبين والمتخصصين. وتشمل حزمة الخدمات الصحية الضرورية المُدرجة في حزمة الخدمات الأساسية خدمات الصحة الإنجابية، وصحة المواليد والأطفال، وبرنامجاً موسعاً للتحصين، والأمراض السارية، والأمراض غير السارية، وخدمات العيادات العامة، والصحة النفسية، والتواصل بهدف تغيير السلوك، والإسعافات الأولية، وصحة الأسنان، والتغذية، وخدمات المختبرات، والخدمات الصيدلانية. وبعض هذه الخدمات أو كلها متوفرة في مراكز الرعاية الصحية الأولية. أما خدمات الرعاية الصحية الأولية التي تُقدِّمها وزارة الصحة فلا تشمل دائماً جميع الخدمات المُدرجة في حزمة الخدمات الصحية الضرورية الكاملة. ولا يزال نقص الأدوية الأساسية، ومحدودية إتاحة الخدمات بسبب ساعات العمل المحدودة، مثاراً للقلق. وتشمل قائمة الأدوية الأساسية، التي وُضِعت في عام 2000، نحو 500 دواء أساسي، منها 210 أدوية لخدمات الرعاية الصحية الأولية. ويوجد رصد محدود لضمان توافق الأدوية الموصوفة مع بروتوكولات العلاج المعمول بها. ويتولى أطباء الأسرة تقديم خدمات ممارسة طب الأسرة، بمساعدة فريق متعدد التخصصات. ويتسم نهج ممارسة طب الأسرة بتقديم خدمات أسرية شاملة ومتواصلة ومتكاملة ومجتمعية المنحى.

التحديات الرئيسية

على الرغم من إدخال تعديلات لتحسين نظام الرعاية الصحية الأولية، توجد تحديات مستمرة تعترض التعزيز المتواصل لجودة الخدمات من خلال ممارسة طب الأسرة. وما زالت هناك فجوات في خدمات طب الأسرة المُخصصة للتوعية الريفية أو لدعم الاحتياجات الصحية للفئات المهمشة في المناطق الريفية أو المناطق المُعرضة للخطر. وتحتاج المشاركة المجتمعية إلى مزيد من التعزيز. ومن أجل تطبيق نموذج ممارسة طب الأسرة، يجري حالياً النظر في إدخال تعديلات على ثلاثة مجالات رئيسية، ألا وهي:2 [1] تحسين صورة وجودة خدمات الرعاية الصحية الأولية وتعزيز العلاقات بين المرضى ومُقدمي الخدمات، [2] توفير خدمات أكثر ملاءمة للمستفيدين، [3] توسيع نطاق نموذج الخدمات وزيادة جودتها. وترتبط هذه العوامل بالتحديات المُحدَّدة التالية عند تطبيق ممارسة طب الأسرة: محدودية ساعات عمل كثيرٍ من مرافق الرعاية الصحية الأولية، عدم وجود نظام شامل لسجلات المرضى، عدم التشديد بما فيه الكفاية على دور الإحالة إلى اختصاصيين أو إلى خدمات أخرى، استمرار احتلال الضفة الغربية وحصار غزة مما يؤدي إلى حدوث نقص مزمن في الأدوية والمعدات.

سُبُل المضيّ قُدُماً

تلتزم وزارة الصحة الفلسطينية التزاماً تاماً بإعادة توجيه نظام الرعاية الصحية الأولية الحالي نحو ممارسة طب الأسرة. وقد تُرجمت هذه الخطوة السياسية إلى إنشاء أول دورة دراسات عليا بشأن طب الأسرة في عام 2010 في الضفة الغربية وفي عام 1990 في غزة.

وتلتزم وزارة الصحة بتطبيق نموذج ممارسة طب الأسرة، بما في ذلك الركائز السبع التالية:2 [1] تكوين فرق مسؤولة عن طب الأسرة، [2] تسجيل المرضى مع فريق مُحدَّد من فرق طب الأسرة، [3] إنشاء سجل إلكتروني واحد للمريض باستخدام رقم هوية وطنية، [4] استحداث نظام مواعيد مصمَّم خصيصاً لتقليل وقت الانتظار وزيادة وقت التواصل مع المريض، [5] تكرار الوصفات الطبية والاستعمال الرشيد للأدوية وتحسين التدبير العلاجي للأمراض غير السارية أو الأمراض المزمنة، [6] الإحالة إلى اختصاصيين أو خدمات أخرى، [7] الرعاية المتكاملة.

المراجع

1. وزارة الصحة الفلسطينية. التقرير السنوي لوزارة الصحة 2016. 2017. قطاع غزة. ص: 68.
2. World Health Organization Towards Family Practice (FP) in Palestine (WHO recommendations for developing a Family Practice Strategy). 2017. Palestine. P. 41.

قطر

مريم علي عبد الملك، زليخة محسن الواحدي، منى طاهر أصيل

26	العدد الإجمالي لمرافق مؤسسة الرعاية الصحية الأولية
220	عدد الممارسين العامّين العاملين في المرافق العامة لمؤسسة الرعاية الصحية الأولية
321	عدد أطباء الأسرة المعتمدين العاملين في مرافق مؤسسة الرعاية الصحية الأولية
8	متوسط عدد خريجي أطباء الأسرة كل سنة
2	عدد كليات الطب
1	عدد أقسام طب الأسرة

مقدمة

تقدم كلٌّ من المرافق العامة والخاصة في قطر خدمات الرعاية الصحية الأولية للمواطنين والمقيمين. وتُعد مؤسسة الرعاية الصحية الأولية أهم وأكبر جهة تُقدم خدمات الرعاية الصحية الأولية في القطاع العام. ويوجد 1.65 مليون مريض مسجل في خدمات مؤسسة الرعاية الصحية الأولية، وقد ثبت أن منهم 1.24 مليون مريض نَشِط. وتتغير هذه القاعدة السكانية باستمرار، ويرجع ذلك في المقام الأول إلى قدوم ورحيل مغتربين يقيمون في قطر مدةً قصيرةً.[1]

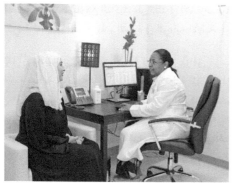

إحدى طبيبات الأسرة مع مريضة في أحد مرافق مؤسسة الرعاية الصحية الأولية

وتركز خدمات الرعاية الصحية الأولية على تعزيز الصحة، والوقاية، والتحري المبكر، والعلاج المستمر للأمراض وتقديم الرعاية. وستصبح هذه الخدمات أكثر تركيزاً على فئات المرضى التي يُطلَق عليها "الفئات السكانية ذات الأولوية" التي تكون في أمسّ الحاجة إلى التركيز على الأطفال والمراهقين، والنساء، والسكان المسنين وكبار السن الأصحاء، والموظفين، ومرضى الصحة النفسية، والمصابين بمرض مزمن.

كما أن مؤسسة الرعاية الصحية الأولية بصدد تطبيق نموذج طب الأسرة الذي سيغير طريقة تقديم المؤسسة للرعاية التي تكون بإشراف طبيب استشاري. ويوفر دليل قطر الوطني للأدوية أداة مرجعية شاملة لإدارة المجموعة المتزايدة من الأدوية المتاحة، وذلك في إطار التوسع الاقتصادي والاجتماعي الشامل في قطر. ويعمل في المؤسسة فرقٌ من الموظفين المتحمسين الذين يتمتعون بدرجة عالية من المهارة في مجال الرعاية الأولية، وينصبُّ تركيزهم على رعاية المرضى والأسر. وجميع مراكز الرعاية الصحية الأولية البالغ عددها 23 مركزاً يديرها أطباء الأسرة بمساعدة فرقٍ متعددة التخصصات. وبدأ تنفيذ برنامج بشأن اعتماد المبادئ التوجيهية السريرية لضمان الحوكمة المناسبة لعملية إعداد هذه المبادئ. وقد أحدثت نُظُم المعلومات السريرية تطوراً ثورياً في مجال الرعاية الأولية من خلال تحسين سلامة وجودة استقاء البيانات والاحتفاظ بها وتسهيل الوصول إلى معلومات المرضى. وانتهت مؤسسة الرعاية الصحية الأولية من المسح الثاني للحصول على الاعتماد الكندي الدولي. وأنشأ قسم البحوث برنامجاً مُعتمَداً بشأن بحوث الموظفين وتدريبهم وبناء قدراتهم من أجل تعزيز القدرات البحثية لدى أطباء الأسرة وغيرهم من موظفي الخطوط الأمامية.

التحديات الرئيسية

يجري حالياً تقييم رسمي للمشروع التجريبي الخاص بممارسة طب الأسرة. وخلال تنفيذ هذا المشروع التجريبي في عام 2017، ظهرت عدة تحديات، كان أهمها[3] التقبُّل الثقافي لزيارة طبيب الأسرة المُعيَّن والحفاظ على استمرارية الرعاية واستمرار النظام الصحي الأوسع نطاقاً في دعم خدمات الرعاية أو الخدمات المتكاملة. وعلى الرغم من التقدم الكبير الذي أحرزته قطر في السنوات الأخيرة، لا يزال النظام الصحي يواجه العديد من التحديات. وجرى تناوُل عدد من التحديات في الاستراتيجيات الصحية الوطنية وكذلك في الخطة الاستراتيجية المؤسسية الخاصة بمؤسسة الرعاية الصحية الأولية للفترة 2018-2022، ألا وهي:[1,2] [1] التغيرات السكانية والخصائص السكانية المعقدة، [2] إحداث تغيير في ثقافة قائمة على علاج الأمراض، [3] الاضطلاع بدور قيادي في الوقاية والرعاية الذاتية، [4] نقص عدد الموظفين على الصعيدين المحلي والعالمي، [5] وتيرة ونطاق التحول في النظام الصحي، [6] مقاومة التغيير وتوقُّعات المرضى المتزايدة باستمرار، [7] الحاجة إلى تعزيز التكامل عبر النظام الصحي.

سُبُل المضيّ قُدُماً

يوجد إصرار واضح على التحول من الرعاية الثانوية إلى الرعاية الأولية، ويتجلى هذا الالتزام الوطني في إنشاء مؤسسة الرعاية الصحية الأولية، وتدعمه الأهداف المُحدَّدة في الاستراتيجية الصحية الوطنية للفترة 2011–2016. وتقدم هذه الاستراتيجية رؤيةً وتوجهاً استراتيجيين شاملين بشأن تقديم الرعاية الصحية، مع تحوُّل واضح من معالجة الأمراض إلى الوقاية وتعزيز الصحة. ويوجد مزيد من التأكيد على ذلك في الاستراتيجية الصحية الوطنية للفترة 2018-2022 [1] بالإضافة إلى مبادرات واضحة مُكرَّسة لتطبيق نموذج طب الأسرة في الرعاية الأولية.

كما أن تطبيق نموذج طب الأسرة في جميع مرافق مؤسسة الرعاية الصحية الأولية توجيةٌ واضح لدى الاستعراض النصفي للاستراتيجية الوطنية للرعاية الصحية الأولية للفترة 2013-2018، وقد التزمت المؤسسة بتطبيق نموذج ممارسة طب الأسرة في المراكز الصحية الجديدة وتحويل جميع المراكز الصحية القائمة إلى هذا النموذج بداية من عام 2018. وسيكون النجاح في تجريب نموذج ممارسة طب الأسرة وتطبيقه وتقييمه مثالاً يُحتذَى به في توحيد خدمات الرعاية الأولية عبر القطاع الصحي. وينبغي فرض اتباع نهج موحَّد لممارسة طب الأسرة في خدمات الرعاية الأولية بجميع مرافق القطاعين العام والخاص مع رصد الأداء والجودة على مستوى وزاري.

المراجع

1. وزارة الصحة العامة. قطر. **الاستراتيجية الوطنية للصحة 2018-2022**. 2018. متاحة على: https://www.moph.gov.qa/ar/HSF/Pages/NHS-18-22.aspx [جرى الاطلاع عليها في 29 آذار/مارس 2018].

2. دائرة إدارة المعلومات الصحية – مؤسسة الرعاية الصحية الأولية في قطر. **تقرير شهر كانون الأول/ديسمبر. التقرير الإحصائي الشهري بشأن إدارة المعلومات الصحية**. 2017.

3. مؤسسة الرعاية الصحية الأولية، فريق مشروع طب الأسرة، 2017.

المملكة العربية السعودية
نهى دشاش، لبنى الأنصاري، إبراهيم الزيق

2400	العدد الإجمالي لمرافق الرعاية الصحية الأولية [1]
6107	عدد الممارسين العامّين العاملين في المرافق العامة للرعاية الصحية الأولية [2]
636	عدد أطباء الأسرة المعتمدين [3] العاملين في مرافق الرعاية الصحية الأولية [2]
100–120	متوسط عدد خريجي أطباء الأسرة (الزمالة والدبلوم) كل سنة [2]
226	إجمالي عدد أطباء الأسرة المقيمين المسجلين في 2015 [2]
25	عدد كليات الطب الحكومية
6	عدد كليات الطب الخاصة [4]
25	عدد أقسام طب الأسرة في كليات الطب [2]
18	عدد برامج طب الأسرة داخل كليات الطب أو برامج الدراسات العليا المشتركة [2]

مقدمة

تغطي شبكة مراكز الرعاية الصحية الأولية معظم السكان، وتوفر رعاية شاملة للمشاكل الصحية الحادة والمزمنة بالإضافة إلى خدمات تعزيز الصحة، مثل التثقيف الصحي والتحصين/التطعيم لجميع المواطنين.[3] ويوجد 2400 مركز للرعاية الصحية الأولية، ويقع 60% منها في مناطق ريفية في جميع أنحاء البلد. ويقوم على تقديم الخدمات 6107 ممارسين عامّين و636 طبيب أسرة. ويقيم معظم أطباء الأسرة في مدن بها أقل من 10% من جميع مراكز الرعاية الصحية الأولية، أما مراكز الرعاية الصحية الأولية الموجودة في مناطق ريفية فيتولى تشغيلها أطباء عامُون. وفي الآونة الأخيرة، شرعت وزارة الصحة في تنفيذ مشروع واسع النطاق لتجديد جميع مباني مراكز الرعاية الصحية الأولية الحكومية، ومن ثَمَّ تحويلها إلى مرافق جذابة حديثة. وتُقدَّم خدمات التصوير بالأشعة في 35% من مراكز الرعاية الصحية الأولية، كما توجد مختبرات في 61% منها.[2]

مريضة تخضع لفحص دوري

والأدوية الأساسية متوفرة في معظم المراكز. وقد تضاعف عدد الأدوية المشمولة خلال السنوات القليلة الماضية لتشمل أكثر من 350 دواءً. وعادةً ما تكون الإحالة بين مراكز الرعاية الصحية الأولية والمستشفيات أقل من المستوى المطلوب.[4] ومن أجل تحسين جودة الرعاية المُقدَّمة في المراكز، وضعت وزارة الصحة برنامجاً مكثفاً بشأن مراقبة الجودة والاعتماد لجميع المراكز. وتستند المبادئ التوجيهية الخاصة بالممارسات السريرية للرعاية الصحية الأولية إلى أدلة بحثية قوية تثبت الفعالية السريرية. وقد أبدى القطاع الخاص رغبته في تقديم خدمات ممارسة طب الأسرة في السنوات القليلة الماضية.

التحديات الرئيسية

تضاربت نتائج الدراسات التي أُجريت لقياس مدى رضا المرضى عن مراكز الرعاية الصحية الأولية. فقد أظهرت دراسة في الرياض[5] أن نحو 30% من المشاركين يرون أن خدمات مركز الرعاية الصحية الأولية ضعيفة أو غير فعالة. وفيما يتعلق باحتمالية اختيار مراكز الرعاية الصحية الأولية بوصفها الخيار الأول للحصول على خدمات الرعاية الصحية، أقر 75% من المشاركين بأن هذه المراكز ليست خيارهم الأول. ولا تزال التغطية الريفية تمثل تحدياً في المملكة العربية السعودية. وأحد

التحديات الرئيسية في تقديم خدمات الرعاية الصحية الأولية المثلى هو الافتقار إلى أطباء أسرة معتمدين. ولا يقتصر هذا النقص على المستوى المحلي، بل هو نقص على المستوى الإقليمي.

سُبُل المضيّ قُدُماً

تشهد المملكة العربية السعودية حالياً إصلاحاً ضخماً. ويهدف هذا التحول إلى تحقيق رؤية 2030 التي وضعها ولي العهد. وسيُسفر التحول في مجال الرعاية الصحية عن نظام مستدام للرعاية الصحية يركز على صحة الناس وعافيتهم. ويتألف هذا النظام من سبعة محاور رئيسية:[5] نموذج الرعاية، وتمويل الرعاية الصحية، وتحويل المؤسسات العامة إلى شركات مساهمة، ومشاركة القطاع الخاص، والحوكمة، والصحة الإلكترونية، والقوى العاملة.

أما جوهر التحول في مجال الرعاية الصحية فيتمثل في نموذج الرعاية الذي يشتمل على ستة نُظُم رعاية، ألا وهي: رعاية الأمراض المزمنة، والولادة الآمنة، والمرحلة الأخيرة، والرعاية المخطط لها، والرعاية العاجلة، والحفاظ على الصحة. وتركز هذه النُّظُم على تفعيل دور الناس والمجتمعات المحلية، مع إيلاء الأولوية للوقاية من الأمراض بوسائل عدة، منها التحرّي وتعزيز الصحة. ويتولى أطباء الأسرة داخل مراكز الرعاية الصحية الأولية تنفيذ قدر كبير من نموذج الرعاية.

ويعتمد هذا النموذج في تقديم الرعاية الصحية على نظام متكامل يُركّز على المريض. وفي الواقع، يدرك قادة الرعاية الصحية في المملكة العربية السعودية أن الطريقة الأكثر فعالية لتوفير رعاية صحية فعالة وعالية الجودة هي من خلال الرعاية الصحية الأولية الفعالة التي يقدمها أطباء الأسرة. وقد شجع ذلك القيادة السياسية على دعم الخطط التي تهدف إلى زيادة عدد أطباء الأسرة المؤهلين والالتزام بتنفيذ هذه الخطط.

المراجع

1. الهيئة العامة للإحصاء مسح الخصائص السكانية. 2017. متاح على: https://www.stats.gov.sa.

2. Al-Khaldi YM, Al-Ghamdi EA, Al-Mogbil TI, Al-Khashan HI. *Family medicine practice in Saudi Arabia: The current situation and proposed strategic directions plan 2020.* Journal of Family and Community Medicine. 2017;24(3): 156–163. doi:10.4103/jfcm.JFCM_41_17.

3. برنامج اعتماد مراكز الرعاية الصحية الأولية. -https://portal.cbahi.gov.sa/english/accreditation- programs/primary-healthcare-center-accreditation-program

4. وزارة التعليم. Moe.gov.sa. 2018 متاح على: https://www.moe.gov.sa (آذار/مارس 2018).

5. Alsakkak MA, Alwahabi SA, Alsalhi HM, Shugdar MA. *Outcome of the first Saudi Central Board for Accreditation of Healthcare Institutions (CBAHI) primary health care accreditation cycle in Saudi Arabia.* Saudi Medical Journal. 2017;38(11): 1132–1136. متاح على: doi:10.15537/smj.2017.11.20760

الصومال
منى أحمد المضواحي، عبد الحميد إبراهيم

457	العدد الإجمالي لمرافق الرعاية الصحية الأولية
1065 في المستشفيات فقط. لا يوجد أطباء يعملون في مرافق الرعاية الصحية الأولية	عدد الممارسين العاميّن العاملين في المرافق العامة للرعاية الصحية الأولية
البيانات غير متوفرة	عدد أطباء الأسرة المعتمدين العاملين في مرافق الرعاية الصحية الأولية
صفر	متوسط عدد خريجي أطباء الأسرة كل سنة
6*	عدد كليات الطب
1 (جامعة بوراما)	عدد أقسام طب الأسرة

* هذه هي كليات الطب المُعترف بها فقط.

مقدمة

تُقدَّم الخدمات الصحية في الصومال من خلال نهج ذي شِقَّين. الشق الأول هو تقديمها من خلال الصندوق الصومالي للمساعدات الإنسانية، الذي كان يُعرف سابقاً باسم الصندوق المشترك للأنشطة الإنسانية، أو خطة الاستجابة الإنسانية التي تهدف إلى تنفيذ عمليات الإغاثة. والشق الثاني هو تقديم الخدمات من خلال حزمة تجريبية وُضعت مؤخراً وجرى تجريبها واعتمادها، تُسمى الحزمة الأساسية للخدمات الصحية، وقد أطلقتها حكومة الصومال الاتحادية في عام 2014 بهدف تحسين الحصول المُنصف على خدمات صحية جيدة ومقبولة بتكلفة ميسورة. وتتوخى هذه العملية الصحية التنموية الارتقاء بمستوى القيادة الحكومية والإدارة والقدرة على تقديم الخدمات، مع الحفاظ على دعم شركاء الصحة، ومن ثَمَّ تجنُّب الفجوة التمويلية الانتقالية التي كثيراً ما

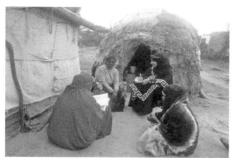
توعية مجتمعية

تحدث خلال فترة ما بعد النزاع، في أثناء انتقال النظام الصحي إلى مرحلة التعافي وإعادة بناء المؤسسات والتنمية.

وقد جرى أيضاً توحيد متطلبات العاملين الصحيين، والأدوية والتكنولوجيات الأساسية اللازمة لتنفيذ تدخلات برامج الحزمة الأساسية للخدمات الصحية. ويتمحور تقديم الخدمات الصحية حول إطار الحزمة الأساسية للخدمات الصحية.[1] ومع ذلك، لا يجري تقديم الخدمات الصحية بشكل موحد في جميع أنحاء البلد، ولا تغطي سوى تسع مناطق من بين 18 منطقة، وذلك بسبب عوامل مثل محدودية الموارد والتحديات الأمنية. أما في المناطق التسع المتبقية، فيتسم تقديم الخدمات الصحية بعدم الاتساق ويعتمد على وجود منظمات إنسانية.

ويشهد القطاع الصحي الخاص في الصومال نمواً سريعاً ويهيمن على تقديم الخدمات الصحية. وتشير الأدلة إلى أن غالبية المرضى يلتمسون المساعدة من القطاع الخاص، مما يدل على صعوبة الوصول إلى المرافق الصحية العامة.

التحديات الرئيسية

يواجه التقديم الفعال للخدمات خمسة تحديات رئيسية: [1] **تمويل الحزمة الأساسية للخدمات الصحية**: تعتمد برامج القطاع الصحي في البلد على الجهات المانحة، وتقل نسبة مساهمة الحكومة عن 2%. [2] **الموارد البشرية الصحية**: القوى العاملة الصحية هي عماد النظام الصحي، وغالباً ما تكون أهم عنصر في تقديم الخدمات الصحية الأساسية المنقذة للحياة

إلى السكان. [3] **مشكلتا انعدام الأمن وتعذُّر الوصول**: تَحدُّ هاتان المشكلتان من قدرة شركاء قطاع الصحة والسلطات على توسيع نطاق الخدمات الصحية وضمان التوزيع العادل للخدمات الصحية. [4] **القدرات المؤسسية وقدرات الحوكمة**: أدى النزاع الذي طال أمده إلى الانهيار التام للنظام الصحي وضعف القدرات المؤسسية. [5] **الإطار التنظيمي لقطاع الصحة**: ساهم ضعف الأطر التنظيمية ومحدودية القدرة على إنفاذ القانون في تدنّي جودة الخدمات الصحية.

سُبُل المضيّ قُدُماً

لتحسين تنفيذ الحزمة الأساسية للخدمات الصحية، لا بد من اتخاذ خمسة إجراءات استراتيجية.[2، 3] **[1] تمويل الحزمة الأساسية للخدمات الصحية تمويلاً مستداماً يمكن التنبؤ به**: يجب على الحكومة زيادة المبالغ المخصصة في الميزانية لتنفيذ الحزمة الأساسية للخدمات الصحية. فالتمويل الخارجي الحالي غير كافٍ، بل غير مستدام أيضاً. [2] **تعزيز توفير قوى عاملة صحية مؤهلة وذات كفاءة في المستوى الوظيفي المتوسط**: إنَّ توفُّر موظفين مؤهلين وأكفاء يمتلكون مزيجاً مناسباً من المهارات أمرٌ محوري لإحياء قطاع الصحة في الصومال. [3] **تعزيز القدرات المؤسسية للسلطات الصحية على جميع المستويات لدعم سيطرة الحكومة ودورها القيادي**: يجب أن يستثمر شركاء التنمية الدوليون الداعمون للقطاع الصحي في بناء القدرات على المستوى الاتحادي ومستوى الولايات والأقاليم لضمان سيطرة الحكومة ودورها القيادي واستدامة برامج قطاع الصحة. [4] **زيادة وضمان الوصول العادل إلى الخدمات الصحية الأساسية وإحراز تقدم نحو تحقيق التغطية الصحية الشاملة**: لكي يحرز البلد تقدماً نحو تحقيق التغطية الصحية الشاملة، ولكي يضمن المساواة في تقديم الخدمات الصحية الأساسية، يجب توسيع نطاق الحزمة الأساسية للخدمات الصحية لتشمل المناطق البدوية والريفية في البلد. [5] **مواصلة إعادة بناء الإطار التنظيمي وتنقيحه لتحسين جودة خدمات الرعاية الصحية والبنية التحتية**: نظراً إلى ضعف المؤسسات العامة والجامعات، يلزم اتباع نهج شراكة شاملة بين القطاعين العام والخاص، مع إطار تنظيمي مُحدَّد جيداً، من أجل تحقيق التغطية الصحية الشاملة في الصومال.

المراجع

1. Pearson N, Muschell J. *Essential Package of Health Services Somaliland 2009.* UNICEF.
متاح على: https://www.unicef.org/somalia/SOM_EssentialSomalilandReport_3_WEB.pdf
2. *World Health Organization.* Strategic review of the Somali Health Sector: Challenges and Prioritized Actions. *Report of the WHO mission to Somalia. September 2015.*
3. *Ministry of Health.* Health Information *Management* System. 2012/13/14.

الفصل 30

السودان

عبد الله سيد أحمد عثمان، إيمان حاج، هند أمين ميرغني، نعيمة القصير

العدد الإجمالي لمرافق الرعاية الصحية الأولية	6220
عدد الممارسين العامّين العاملين في المرافق العامة للرعاية الصحية الأولية	غير متاح
عدد أطباء الأسرة المعتمدين العاملين في مرافق الرعاية الصحية الأولية	46
متوسط عدد خريجي أطباء الأسرة كل سنة	40 طبيباً، و300 من الحاصلين على الماجستير
عدد كليات الطب	37
عدد أقسام طب الأسرة	5

مقدمة

تتصدر الرعاية الصحية الأولية أجندة الإصلاح المستمر للنظام الصحي في السودان. وتشير التقارير إلى أن نسبة التغطية بالرعاية الصحية الأولية في الوقت الحالي تبلغ 95% من السكان. ولكن يُحرَز تقدُّم أقل في التغطية التي تقوم بها مراكز ووحدات صحة الأسرة العاملة، إذ كانت التغطية بحلول منتصف عام 2017 تبلغ 88% من السكان في حالة المراكز و77% من السكان في حالة الوحدات. ومع زيادة الالتزام الحكومي والتمويل المستدام، يجري توسيع نطاق تغطية الرعاية الصحية الأولية ليشمل فئات سكانية محرومة. وجاء في تقرير التقييم المشترك لعام 2017 أن ثلاث ولايات، هي القضارف وسنار ونهر النيل، أفادت بتحقيق وحدات صحة الأسرة لجميع مهامها الوظيفية، بينما أبلغت ولايتا البحر الأحمر وجنوب كردفان عن تحقيق وحدات صحة الأسرة لأقل من 50% من أدائها الوظيفي، وأبلغت ولايتان أخريان، هما شمال دارفور ووسط دارفور، عن تحقيق الوحدات لأقل من 50% من أدائها الوظيفي.1

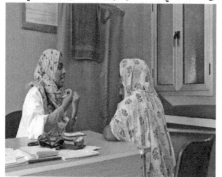

طبيبة الرعاية الصحية الأولية مع مريضة

وتتسم حزم الخدمات الصحية الأساسية بأنها مُجزَّأة وتختلف من مُقدِّم خدمات إلى آخر. وتقضي سياسة التمويل الصحي الخاصة بوزارة الصحة بالفصل بين مُقدِّم الخدمة ومشتريها.2

وقد حظيت البنية التحتية للرعاية الصحية الأولية باهتمام كبير من جانب وزارة الصحة في السنوات الأخيرة. ولقد بدأ في عام 2012 تنفيذ مشروع توسيع، يركز في المقام الأول على البنية التحتية وتدريب الموارد البشرية الصحية. أما محتوى حزمة الخدمات الصحية الأساسية المُقدَّمة على مستوى الرعاية الصحية الأولية فيتوقف على عبء الأمراض. وتضمن السياسة التمويلية قيام الصندوق الوطني للتأمين الصحي بتقديم حزمة الخدمات الصحية الأساسية والحزمة الشاملة إلى جميع السكان المؤمَّن عليهم بالإضافة إلى الفقراء.2 وقد ارتفعت نسبة المرافق الصحية التي تقدم حزمة الخدمات الصحية الأساسية الكاملة من 24% إلى 62% بين عامي 2011 و2016. 3 كما أثبتت دراسة حديثة أن نسبة توفر الأدوية الأساسية بلغت 73% في المرافق الصحية العامة و90% في المرافق الصحية الخاصة.4

كما أن بروتوكولات العلاج والمبادئ التوجيهية ليست موحدة ولا تُنفَّذ بالكامل. وقد بُذلت عدة جهود لتعزيز نظام الإحالة. ويُجرى حالياً إصلاح في المعلومات الصحية لتحقيق مزيد من التكامل، كما أُنشئ مجلس اعتماد.

التحديات

يتمثل أحد أكبر التحديات في أن غالبية خريجي أطباء الأسرة يهاجرون إلى دول في منطقة الخليج وغيرها، ولا يتبقى منهم في البلد لممارسة هذه المهنة سوى عدد ضئيل.4 ورغم أن أحد الأهداف الثلاثة الرئيسية التي يسعى إليها مشروع توسيع الرعاية الصحية الأولية هو ضمان جودة واستدامة خدمات الرعاية الصحية الأولية، إلا أنه لا يوجد نظام يعمل بشكل جيد لضمان الجودة، ويوجد نقص في البروتوكولات السريرية والمبادئ التوجيهية ومعايير الجودة والمؤشرات. ومن ناحية أخرى، طُبِّقت بعض الاستراتيجيات والأنشطة لتحسين جودة خدمات الرعاية الصحية الأولية، مثل معايير بناء وإصلاح البنية التحتية ومعدات المرافق الصحية، بالإضافة إلى توظيف وتدريب أطباء الأسرة وأعضاء فرق الصحة الأسرية.3

سُبُل المضيّ قُدُماً

تتمثل أولوية الصندوق الوطني للتأمين الصحي خلال السنوات القادمة في شمول جميع الفقراء بالإعانات الحكومية. ونجحت الحكومة في توسيع نطاق التغطية الصحية للفقراء فارتفع عدد الأسر المشمولة من 500 ألف أسرة إلى 750 ألف أسرة ثم إلى مليون أسرة خلال السنوات الثلاث الماضية. وعلاوة على ذلك، وُضعت مبادئ توجيهية بشأن الشراء، كآلية لتعزيز التنفيذ. كما يتصدر مشروع توسيع نطاق الرعاية الصحية الأولية جدول أعمال الحكومة، وتموّله وزارة المالية. وقد ازداد على المستوى الوطني الالتزام السياسي بممارسة طب الأسرة خلال السنوات الأخيرة. ويُعدّ المجلس القومي لتنسيق الخدمات الصحية، الذي يرأسه رئيس دولة السودان، أعلى سلطة صحية في السودان. ويلتزم هذا المجلس بتحقيق التغطية الصحية الشاملة، وقد أقرَّ سياسة صحة الأسرة. وتعمل وزارة الصحة على تحقيق التغطية الصحية الشاملة، وتطبيق نهج صحة الأسرة، من خلال توسيع نطاق الرعاية الصحية الأولية وتدريب الأطباء في مجال طب الأسرة فضلاً عن الموظفين الصحيين الآخرين.3، 5 ولسياسة صحة الأسرة ثلاثة أهداف رئيسية، ألا وهي: [1] تعزيز نظام تقديم خدمات الرعاية الصحية الأولية من أجل تقديم خدمات صحية جيدة تتسم بالكفاءة والإنصاف، [2] تحسين الاعتراف بتخصص طب الأسرة، وزيادة استبقاء أطباء الأسرة، [3] ضمان تخرج أطباء أسرة أكُفاء وعاملين صحيين مساعدين من أجل تقديم خدمات صحية متكاملة محورها الإنسان على مستوى الرعاية الصحية الأولية.6

المراجع

1. وزارة الصحة الاتحادية. تقرير التقييم المشترك، السودان 2017.
2. وزارة الصحة الاتحادية، معهد الصحة العامة. سياسة التمويل الصحي. 2015.
3. وزارة الصحة الاتحادية، معهد الصحة العامة طب الأسرة في السودان: تحليل للوضع الراهن. 2015.
4. وزارة الصحة الاتحادية، معهد الصحة العامة. السياسة الصحية الوطنية 2017-2030.
5. وزارة الصحة الاتحادية، الإدارة العامة للرعاية الصحية الأولية، مشروع التوسيع. التقرير السنوي لعام 2017.
6. وزارة الصحة الاتحادية. تعزيز الرعاية الصحية الأولية في السودان من خلال نهج صحة الأسرة: خيارات السياسات. 2016.

سوريا

ماجد البيطار، أروى عيسى

1826	عدد مرافق الرعاية الصحية الأولية
850	عدد الممارسين العامّين العاملين في المرافق العامة للرعاية الصحية الأولية
100	عدد أطباء الأسرة المتخصصين العاملين في مرافق الرعاية الصحية الأولية
8	*متوسط عدد خريجي أطباء الأسرة كل سنة*
8	*عدد الجامعات الطبية أو كليات الطب*
2	*عدد شُعب أو أقسام طب الأسرة*

مقدمة

لا شكّ في أن الأزمة التي مرّت بها سوريا خلال السنوات السبع الماضية قد أثّرت في قطاع الصحة. فقد تعرضت مستشفيات ومراكز صحية كثيرة لأضرار هيكلية على نحو كليّ أو جزئي. وتوقف بعضها تماماً عن العمل، وقلّص البعض الآخر خدماته أو اضطُرّ إلى استخدام مبانٍ مجاورة لتقديم الخدمات. وإضافةً إلى ذلك، تعطلت الشبكات العامة للكهرباء والمياه تعطلاً شبه دائم في أغلب الأحيان. وأصبح كثير من سيارات وزارة الصحة، لا سيما سيارات الإسعاف، غير صالح للعمل، بسبب استهدافها المباشر أو غير المباشر.

وتقلّص بشدة عدد المهنيين الصحيين.[1] وتشمل التحديات صعوبة الحصول على مياه نظيفة؛ وتعطُّل شبكات الصرف الصحي؛ والاكتظاظ خاصة في أماكن الإيواء، نتيجةً لوصول سكان نازحين من أماكن غير آمنة؛ وانعدام الأمن الغذائي بدرجات متفاوتة؛ وزيادة الضغط على ما تبقى من المراكز الصحية العاملة.

مركز نوى الأول لصحة الأسرة، بمدينة درعا

وإضافةً إلى ذلك، تضاعف عدد الذين يعانون الضائقة النفسية والاكتئاب والإدمان والأمراض النفسية الخطيرة، فضلاً عن تضاعف عدد حالات الانتحار. وأدى ذلك إلى تدهور الوضع الصحي في البلد تدهوراً خطيراً. وتضاءلت معدلات التغطية بالتطعيم، وسُجِّلت حالات متعددة مصابة بسوء التغذية، وظهر شلل الأطفال والحصبة وغيرهما من الأمراض، لا سيما الأمراض السارية.[2] ويجري بانتظام تحديث قائمة الأدوية الأساسية واستعراضها. وبروتوكولات العلاج ليست متاحة للجميع في المراكز الصحية. كما أن نظام الإحالة غير مُستخدَم حالياً. ونظام معلومات الرعاية الصحية الأولية هو نظام المعلومات الصحية الروتينية. ويزداد يوماً بعد يوم دور القطاع الخاص في توفير خدمات العيادات الخارجية.

التحديات

تواجه عملية إتاحة خدمات جيدة التحديات الجسيمة التالية:[3] [1] توقُّف كثير من المراكز الصحية عن العمل تماماً، بالإضافة إلى تضرُّر كثير من المراكز الأخرى تضرراً جزئياً، مع وجود حاجة ماسة إلى إصلاحها، [2] ضعف القدرات والموارد، وما يترتب على ذلك من تأثير على جاهزية المراكز وجودة الخدمات، [3] تضاعُف عدد زوار بعض المراكز نتيجةً لانتقال السكان إلى أماكن أكثر أمناً، مما جعل من الصعب تقديم خدمات عادلة وجيدة لجميع المرضى، [4] عدم تدريب مَن ينوبون عن الأشخاص الذين يؤدون خدمات معينة في بعض المراكز الصحية. وتشمل التحديات التي تواجه ممارسة طب الأسرة ما يلي: [1] الافتقار إلى قرارات سياسية داعمة، [2] عدم دعم وزارة الصحة لاختصاصيي طب الأسرة، [3] غياب الحافز الكافي لأطباء الأسرة الماهرين، والحاجة إلى العمل في عيادات خاصة بجانب العمل في مرافق الرعاية الصحية، [4] الافتقار إلى مبادرات عامة أو

خاصة للتمكين من ممارسة طب الأسرة أو التشجيع على ممارسته.

سُبُل المضيّ قُدُماً

إن تقديم خدمات صحية متكاملة في ظل أزمة طويلة الأمد له تأثير كبير على قطاع الصحة، لا سيما على مرافق الرعاية الصحية الأولية. وقد كانت الأولوية، ولا تزال، تُمنَح لاستعادة الخدمات الأساسية، وإصلاح المراكز المتضررة وترميمها، وتوفير الكوادر البشرية وإعادة توزيعها، وإعادة جميع معدلات التغطية الصحية إلى ما كانت عليه قبل الأزمة. وقد واصلت وزارة الصحة تقديم خدمات الرعاية الصحية الأولية الأساسية حتى في الأماكن التي يصعب الوصول إليها وتخرج عن نطاق السيطرة. وعلاوة على ذلك، اضطلعت الوزارة، ولا تزال تضطلع، بحملات تطعيم وطنية نشِطة. ووفرت الوزارة أماكن إيواء في جميع المحافظات والأقاليم، بالإضافة إلى توفير الطاقم الطبي الضروري والأدوية اللازمة وإمكانية إحالة الحالات الحرجة. وقد وضعت الوزارة، منذ بداية الأزمة، خطة استراتيجية لتقديم خدمات الصحة النفسية والرعاية النفسية الأولية من خلال مراكز مُختارة من مراكز الرعاية الصحية الأولية. ومن أجل تقييم الوضع الحالي وتحديث البيانات الخاصة بتقييم وجاهزية الخدمات الصحية المُقدَّمة في جميع المراكز الصحية، تُجرى حالياً «دراسة استقصائية لتقييم مدى توفر الخدمات وجاهزتها» بالتعاون مع منظمة الصحة العالمية. ويجري العمل منذ أكثر من عامين على إصلاح المراكز الصحية وترميمها. وقد أوْلَت وزارة الصحة اهتماماً كبيراً لمسألة مكافحة العدوى من خلال التنسيق والتعاون مع السلطات المعنية.

المراجع

1. Statistical Memorandum of the Directorate of Planning and International Cooperation (2017). متاح على: /http://www.moh.gov.sy
2. Epidemiological Bulletins of the WHO for Early Warning Alert and Response System, for the 2017 year. متاح على: http://www.emro.who.int/syr/ewars-workshops/ewars-bulletins-2017.html.
3. Regulatory Decision No T/8 (Oct 2017), Integrated Health Centers (Health Centers-Specialized Health Centers), [supplement No 1: Human Resources].

تونس
علي مطيراوي، بلقاسم صبري

العدد الإجمالي لمرافق الرعاية الصحية الأولية	2091
عدد الممارسين العامّين العاملين في المرافق العامة للرعاية الصحية الأولية	5000
عدد أطباء الأسرة المعتمدين العاملين في مرافق الرعاية الصحية الأولية	150
متوسط عدد خريجي أطباء الأسرة كل سنة	80
عدد كليات الطب	4
عدد أقسام طب الأسرة	4

مقدمة

حقَّق نظام الرعاية الصحية التونسي مؤشرات صحية جيدة من حيث العمر المتوقع المتوقع وانخفاض الوفيات والمراضة، وهو يباري البلدان المشابهة في الدخل ومستوى الإنفاق على الرعاية الصحية داخل إقليم شرق المتوسط وخارجه[1].

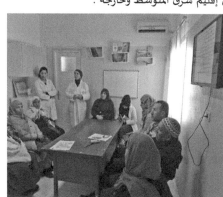

وترجع أيضاً الإنجازات الصحية إلى تحسين المُحدِّدات الاجتماعية للصحة، بما في ذلك التعليم وحقوق المرأة، والحماية الصحية الاجتماعية الواسعة النطاق منذ استقلال تونس في أواخر خمسينيات القرن العشرين.

وقد أتاحت السياسة السكانية الجريئة التي اعتُمدت في منتصف الستينيات دمج تنظيم الأسرة والصحة الإنجابية في مواقع الرعاية الصحية الأولية، وساعدت هذه السياسة على التحكم في النمو السكاني.

برنامج صحة المجتمع

ويتمتع نظام الرعاية الصحية بشبكة قوية من مرافق الرعاية الأولية في كلٍّ من القطاعين العام والخاص، ويركز هذا النظام على تعزيز الصحة والوقاية. كما أن ما يقرب من 50% من الأطباء ممارسون عامُّون يعملون في فرق صحية في القطاع العام، ويشتركون في تقديم الرعاية التعزيزية والوقائية والعلاجية والتأهيلية والمُلطِّفة من خلال برامج وطنية تديرها وزارة الصحة.

أما في القطاع الخاص، فيعمل الممارسون العامُّون في عيادات فردية خاصة، ويقدمون فيها الرعاية العلاجية في المقام الأول، ولا يشاركون مشاركة كاملة في البرامج الوطنية لتعزيز الصحة والوقاية على الرغم من الجهود المبذولة من خلال التثقيف الصحي وفرص مواصلة التطوير المهني.

التحديات

يواجه النظام الصحي التونسي تحديات كبيرة، منها التحولات الوبائية والديمغرافية المتقدمة، وتدهوُر كثيرٍ من المُحدِّدات الاجتماعية للصحة، وتزايد توقعات السكان بشأن الحصول على رعاية صحية جيدة في حين أن الموارد آخِذة في التناقص.

وتتزايد عوامل الخطر يوماً بعد يوم، ومنها ارتفاع معدل انتشار التدخين وتعاطي المخدرات، والبدانة، وقلة النشاط البدني، والنظام الغذائي غير المناسب خاصة بين الشباب، وحوادث الطرق، والعنف المنزلي. ويؤدي هذا الوضع إلى زيادة الضغوط الاقتصادية وضغوط تقديم الخدمات التي يتعرض لها النظام الصحي بسبب زيادة الأمراض المزمنة وغير السارية.

ويجب أن تصبح الخدمات المُقدَّمة أكثر مواءمة للمجتمع المحلي مع التركيز على تعزيز أنماط الحياة الصحية وعلى تحسين المحددات الاجتماعية الرئيسية للصحة. ولا يزال التعاون مع منظمات المجتمع المدني والتنسيق مع القطاعات الأخرى ذات الصلة محدوداً، رغم الجهود التي بُذلت بعد ثورة 2011[2].

ولقد كان للقيود المالية، الناتجة عن برامج التكيُّف الهيكلي التي بدأت منذ أواخر ثمانينيات القرن العشرين، تأثيرٌ سلبيٌّ على توفُّر التقنيات الصحية والقوى العاملة المطلوبة في مواقع الرعاية الصحية الأولية. كما تتناقص يوماً بعد يوم فرص مواصلة التعليم والتطوير المهني المتاحة للموظفين العاملين في مرافق الخط الأول.

سُبُل المضيّ قُدُماً

هناك فرص يتيحها دستور الدولة الجديد الذي يحمي الحق في الصحة والالتزام السياسي بالتغطية الصحية الشاملة من خلال الرعاية الصحية الأولية التي تركز على المجتمع. وقد صدر قانون بشأن تطوير إصلاح طب الأسرة بدأ تطبيقُه في عام 2017.

ويشتمل إصلاح طب الأسرة على تغييرات في المقررات الدراسية للدراسات الطبية الجامعية، وإعداد تدريب خاص، وإعادة تدريب الممارسين العامّين العاملين في القطاعين العام والخاص تدريجياً. ويجري حالياً الإعداد لإنشاء فروع لمؤسسات تعليمية أجنبية داخل تونس من أجل دعم تدريب فرق صحة الأسرة باستخدام الشبكة المهمة لمرافق الخط الأول. ويجري تعزيز المسؤوليات الاجتماعية لكليات الطب من خلال التركيز على النهوض بالصحة والحماية.

وتُجرى حالياً مفاوضات بشأن حوافز مالية وغير مالية، منها الاعتراف بتخصص طب الأسرة، بين وزارات الصحة وكليات الطب ووزارة التعليم العالي. ومن المزمع بذل جهود لتحسين ظروف عمل الفِرق الصحية العاملة في الرعاية الأولية، وللسعي إلى زيادة المشاركة الفعالة للمجتمع وتمكينه.

المراجع

1. Mtiraoui A, Gueddana N. The family and reproductive health program in underprivileged areas in Tunisia; *Actes CICRED Seminar on Reproductive Health, Unmet Needs and Poverty: Issues of Access and Quality of Services*, Bangkok 25-30 November 2002, pp 11.

2. Forum national sur la santé. Rapport de synthèse du groupe de travail sur les déterminants de la santé. 1997. متاح على: http://www.hc-sc.gc.ca/hcs-sss/pubs/care-soins/1997-nfoh-fnss-v2/legacy_heritage4_f.html

الإمارات العربية المتحدة

هيفاء حمد فارس العلي، وديعة محمد الشريف

العدد الإجمالي لمرافق الرعاية الصحية الأولية	131
عدد الممارسين العامّين العاملين في المرافق العامة للرعاية الصحية الأولية	968
عدد أطباء الأسرة المعتمدين العاملين في مرافق الرعاية الصحية الأولية	382
متوسط عدد خريجي أطباء الأسرة كل سنة	25
عدد كليات الطب	6
عدد أقسام طب الأسرة	6

مقدمة

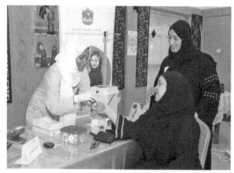

التحرّي والتوعية

يشهد قطاع الرعاية الصحية في دولة الإمارات العربية المتحدة اشتراك جهات عامة وخاصة في تقديم خدمات الرعاية الصحية. أما خدمات الرعاية الصحية العامة فتُديرها وتُنظمها وزارة الصحة والوقاية، وهيئات حكومية محلية مثل دائرة الصحة في أبو ظبي، وشركة أبو ظبي للخدمات الصحية، وهيئة الصحة بدبي. وتنص رؤية الإمارات 2021، التي تتوافق تماماً مع أهداف الأمم المتحدة للتنمية المستدامة، على أن "دولة الإمارات [سوف]. تستثمر باستمرار في مجال الرعاية الصحية لتشييد بنية تحتية بمعايير عالمية، وتوفير الخبرات والخدمات اللازمة لتلبية احتياجات المواطنين وتوقعاتهم المتزايدة".[1] وتهدف هذه الرؤية إلى الارتقاء بمستوى الرعاية الصحية من خلال اعتماد جميع المرافق الصحية بحلول عام 2021. كما تهدف إلى الحد من الأمراض غير السارية وزيادة أنماط الحياة الصحية في المجتمع. ولتحقيق هذه الرؤية، وضعت الحكومة أجندة وطنية ذات مؤشرات قابلة للقياس. وتركز الرعاية الصحية الأولية على طب الأسرة بوصفه تخصصاً طبياً يوفر الرعاية الصحية المستمرة والمتكاملة والشاملة للأفراد والأسر.

ولقد حققت دولة الإمارات تقدماً ملحوظاً في جميع مؤشرات صحة الأمهات والأطفال.[2, 3] ويوفر نموذج عيادة الأمراض غير السارية ضمن الرعاية الصحية الأولية رعاية متكاملة من أجل الوقاية من الأمراض ومكافحتها وعلاجها لمرضى السكري، وارتفاع ضغط الدم، وعسر شحميات الدم، والأمراض الرئوية المزمنة، والأمراض النفسية. ويُعد برنامج الصحة المدرسية أحد برامج الرعاية الصحية الأولية الرائدة التي تقدم خدمات وقائية وتعزيزية وعلاجية. كما أن خدمات إسداء المشورة بشأن الإقلاع عن التدخين في الرعاية الأولية تحفز وتساعد المدخنين على الإقلاع عن التدخين. ويعمل حالياً في القطاع العام 382 طبيب أسرة معتمداً. ويخضع جميع العاملين في الرعاية الصحية الأولية المُعيَّنين حديثاً لبرنامج تدريبي قائم على الكفاءة. وتستخدم 85% من مراكز الرعاية الصحية الأولية سجلات صحية إلكترونية. وطرحت الحكومة تطبيقاً يوفر للمرضى بوابة إلكترونية ذكية ويسمح لهم بالاطلاع على سجلاتهم. وحصل 60% من مراكز الرعاية الأولية العامة على اعتماد اللجنة الدولية المشتركة لاعتماد المنشآت الصحية (JCIA)، ومن المستهدف أن تصل نسبة المراكز الحاصلة على هذا الاعتماد إلى 100% بحلول عام 2021.

التحديات الرئيسية

[1] تُعتبر **تنمية القوى العاملة** من المجالات التي تتطلب نمواً كبيراً ومستداماً. فنسبة المُمرضين الإماراتيين لا تتجاوز 3%، ويتخرج 25 طبيب أسرة في المتوسط كل عام. [2] **يمثل التحول السكاني** الذي سيضاعف نسبة الإماراتيين الذين تزيد

أعمارهم عن 60 عاماً بحلول عام 2032 تحدياً كبيراً لتحسين رعاية المسنين في دولة الإمارات. [3] **يؤدي ارتفاع معدلات انتشار أمراض القلب والأوعية الدموية، والسمنة، والسكري** إلى زيادة عبء الرعاية الصحية. وتدرك الحكومة هذه المشاكل جيداً، وتتخذ إجراءات جيدة التنظيم في إطار الأجندة الوطنية. [4] **نشاط البحوث الطبية** المتعلقة بالرعاية الأولية، محدود في دولة الإمارات. [5] مع التطور الهائل في قطاع الرعاية الصحية الخاص، يوجد حالياً إفراط في استخدام أنواع معينة من الخدمات، مما يزيد التكاليف ويقلل الكفاءة.

سُبُل المضيّ قُدُماً

من مشروعات تحسين النظام الصحي مبادرة "بيتنا الطبي" للرعاية الصحية الأولية التي أطلقتها الخدمات العلاجية الخارجية التابعة لشركة أبو ظبي للخدمات الصحية، وهي نموذج رعاية قائم على مبادئ طب الأسرة. ويعتمد هذا النموذج على تعزيز الحصول على الخدمات، والتفاعل بين المريض ومُقدِّم الخدمة الشخصي، والإدارة الذاتية. فالمريض المُسجَّل في أي مركز من مراكز الرعاية الأولية سيَعتبر المركزَ بيتَه الطبي. وسيكون طبيب الرعاية الأولية، بصفته مُقدِّم الرعاية الأولية، مسؤولاً عن تلبية احتياجات المريض الحالية والمستقبلية. ولقد جرى توفير ونشْر عيادات متنقلة لخدمة المناطق النائية في إمارة أبو ظبي التي تواجه صعوبة في الوصول إلى مرافق الرعاية الصحية، ولتقديم خدمات الرعاية الصحية في المناسبات العامة ومواقع العمل والمدارس. وفي عام 2016، قدمت وزارة الصحة أيضاً عيادة صحية متنقلة. وأُنشِئت وحدة لرعاية المسنين، تتألف من فريق متعدد التخصصات يضم طبيباً متخصصاً في أمراض الشيخوخة، وطبيباً متخصصاً في طب الأسرة، وطبيباً متخصصاً في الطب المجتمعي، وطبيباً فيزيائياً، واختصاصي علاج طبيعي، وممرضات، ومرشداً اجتماعياً، واختصاصي تغذية.

المراجع

1. رؤية الإمارات 2021، الأجندة الوطنية. متاحة على: https://www.vision2021.ae/en [جرى الاطلاع عليها في: 9 كانون الثاني/يناير 2019].
2. UAE Demographics Profile 2017. متاح على: https://www.indexmundi.com/united_arab_emirates/demographics_profile.html [جرى الاطلاع عليه في: 9 كانون الثاني/يناير 2019].
3. World Health Organization. *WHO Vaccine-Preventable Diseases: Monitoring System. 2018 Global Summary.* متاح على: http://apps.who.int/immunization_monitoring/globalsummary/countries?countrycriteria%5Bcountry%5D%5B%5D=ARE&commit=OK [جرى الاطلاع عليه في: 9 كانون الثاني/يناير 2019].

اليمن

علي المضواحي

العدد الإجمالي لمرافق الرعاية الصحية الأولية	إجمالي المرافق الصحية: 4602 أخرى: 3
عدد الممارسين العامّين العاملين في المرافق العامة للرعاية الصحية الأولية	2389
عدد أطباء الأسرة المعتمدين العاملين في مرافق الرعاية الصحية الأولية	3
متوسط عدد خريجي أطباء الأسرة كل سنة	6
عدد كليات الطب	9
عدد أقسام طب الأسرة	3

المستشفيات: 255، المراكز الصحية: 1055، الوحدات الصحية: 3289

مقدمة

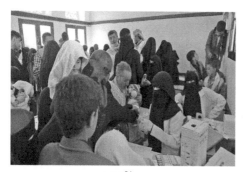

حملة تمنيع

لقد خلَّفت الحرب الدائرة في اليمن 18.8 مليون شخص في حاجة إلى مساعدات إنسانية، وألقت عبئاً هائلاً على النظام الصحي اليمني في وقت تشتد فيه الحاجة إلى هذا النظام. وهناك ما يقرب من 7 ملايين شخص في حاجة ماسة إلى الغذاء، ومستويات سوء التغذية آخِذة في الارتفاع، مما يضع البلد على حافة المجاعة. ويعاني نحو 462 ألف طفل من سوء التغذية الحاد الوخيم مع احتمالية حدوث مضاعفات تهدد الحياة. وتقل نسبة المرافق الصحية التي تعمل بكامل طاقتها عن 45%، فهناك 274 مرفقاً على الأقل تعرَّض للضرر أو الدمار خلال النزاع الحالي الذي بدأ في آذار/مارس 2015. [1] كما أُرغم العاملون في مجال الرعاية الصحية على الرحيل إلى أماكن أخرى، والذين لا يزالون يعملون منهم لا يتلقَّوْن رواتبهم بانتظام.

وبدعم من التحالف العالمي لِلِّقاحات، شرعت وزارة الصحة العامة والسكان في اتباع نهج متكامل في تقديم الخدمات الصحية الأساسية، باستخدام المرافق الثابتة وجلسات التوعية. وكان النظام الصحي المحلي يمثل الأساس الذي استُند إليه في وضع نموذج التكامل. وانخفض معدل وفيات الأطفال دون سن الخامسة بنسبة 50% تقريباً من 102 في عام 2003 إلى 51 في عام 2013، كما انخفض معدل وفيات الأمهات من 365 إلى 148 خلال الفترة نفسها. وشرعت وزارة الصحة العامة والسكان مؤخراً في تنفيذ حزمة الحد الأدنى من الخدمات، بدعم من منظمة الصحة العالمية. وفي الفترة ما بين عامي 2006 و2010، أعدت الوزارة أدلة تدريب، ومبادئ توجيهية، وسياسات تقديم الخدمات المتكاملة.

وتُعدّ إمكانية تحقيق التغطية الصحية الشاملة محدودة بسبب صعوبة الحصول على الرعاية الصحية والعوائق المالية[2]. وكان آخر تحديث لقائمة الأدوية الأساسية في عام 2014، وتحتوي هذه القائمة على 437 دواءً. وجاء اليمن في المرتبة رقم 160 من أصل 188 بلداً حسب مؤشر التنمية البشرية. ويحتل المرتبة الأخيرة من بين 155 بلداً مدرجاً في مؤشر عدم المساواة بين الجنسين. كما أن أعداد الموظفين الصحيين المؤهلين في المناطق الريفية غير كافية، ولقد أجبرت الحرب كثيراً منهم على الفرار من ديارهم.

التحديات الرئيسية

أكثر أسباب الوفاة شيوعاً هي عدوى الجهاز التنفسي السفلي (28%)، ومرض القلب الإقفاري (9.5%)، والسكتة الدماغية (6.8%)، ومضاعفات الولادة المبتسرة (6.6%)، والإصابات الناجمة عن حوادث المرور (3.8%).[3] وعلى الرغم من الجهود المبذولة للحد من ارتفاع معدلات وفيات الأمهات والأطفال دون سن الخامسة، فلا يزال سوء التغذية من المشكلات الصحية الرئيسية. وقد سبق أن سُجِّلت مستويات مرتفعة من التقزم ونقص الوزن والهزال في مسح الصحة الأسرية لعام 2003، قبل الحرب.[4] ونظراً إلى التحديات الهائلة التي يواجهها اليمن، تقف ممارسة طب الأسرة حالياً في مفترق طرق من حيث تنفيذها. فالتحديات الأمنية والطلب المتزايد على رعاية الإصابات الشديدة أضعفَا من قدرة ممارسة طب الأسرة على الوفاء بوعودها. ولا يستطيع مقدمو الرعاية الصحية أداء واجباتهم على النحو الأمثل بسبب الأزمات السياسية والاقتصادية المستمرة.

سُبُل المضيّ قُدُماً

في إطار تعزيز النظام الصحي الوطني، اعتمدت وزارة الصحة العامة والسكان نهج رعاية يُركِّز على الأسرة. وأنشأت الوزارة إدارة عامة لصحة الأسرة، يرأسُها نائب وزير، وتعمل هذه الإدارة على اتباع نهج متكامل في اتخاذ القرارات المتعلقة بالرعاية الصحية داخل قطاع الرعاية الصحية الأولية. وكانت إدارة صحة الأسرة التابعة لوزارة الصحة العامة والسكان قد نجحت، قبل آذار/مارس 2015، في قيادة تدخلات الرعاية الصحية الأولية المتكاملة من خلال مرافق الرعاية الصحية الأولية وأنشطة التوعية. وقد ظهر بوضوح التركيز على برامج الصحة العامة الأساسية على المستوى المحلي، من خلال برامج بناء القدرات التي عزَّزت تقديم الخدمات الصحية الأساسية. وأسفر النهج المتكامل لخدمات الرعاية الصحية الأولية عن تحسينات كبيرة في صحة الأمهات والأطفال. وما فتئ هذا التحسن يتراجع منذ اندلاع الحرب في آذار/مارس 2015. وترى وزارة الصحة العامة والسكان أن القطاع الخاص شريك تنموي محتمل يمكن التعاقد معه لتوفير التغطية في مجالات لا يستطيع القطاع العام توفير التغطية فيها، لا سيما في مجال التحصين وخدمات الصحة الإنجابية.

المراجع

1. WHO, Health Resources Availability Mapping System (HeRAMS), Yemen, 2017.
2. MoPHP. Yemen. *NHS 2010-2025. 2010.* متاح على: http://www.nationalplanningcycles.org/sites/default/files/planning_cycle_repository/yemen/nat_health_strategy_-_yemen_eng.pdf [جرى الاطلاع عليه في 24 نيسان/أبريل 2018].
3. *The Health Cluster Response Strategy to Yemen's Crisis for 2015-2016, Yemen, October 2015.*
4. MoPHP, Yemen. *Family Health Survey, Yemen, 2003.*